INDEPENDENCE WITHOUT SIGHT OR SOUND

Suggestions for Practitioners Working with Deaf-Blind Adults

DONA SAUERBURGER

AFB
American Foundation for the Blind
New York

97 96 95 94 93 5 4 3 2 1

Printed in the United States of America

Library of Congress Cataloging-in-Publication Data

Sauerburger, Dona, 1946-
Independence without sight or sound: suggestions for practitioners working with deaf-blind adults / Dona Sauerburger.
p. cm.
Includes bibliographical references (p.) and index.
ISBN 0-89128-246-7
1. Blind-deaf—Education. 2. Blind-deaf—Means of communication.
I. Title.
HV1597.2.S28 1993 92-47348
362.4'186—dc20 CIP

Photo credits: J. David Carrigan, pages 51, 53 (bottom), 54, 55, 56, 57; Jenna R. Herron, cover and pages 18, 46; Suzanne Jones, page 53 (top); Dona Sauerburger, pages 68, 76, 123; Frederick J. Sauerburger, pages 62, 106; Mark F. Sauerburger, page 52.

CONTENTS

FOREWORD

In *Independence Without Sight or Sound,* Dona Sauerburger has provided us with a vivid picture of what it means to have limited access to the world around us. But she has also provided us with a wealth of insights, strategies, and techniques for how to communicate and feel comfortable with our deaf-blind clients, colleagues, and acquaintances. As an orientation and mobility (O&M) instructor with more than 20 years of experience, she has shared an extraordinary amount of useful information that O&M instructors, rehabilitation teachers and counselors, interpreters, employers, and families will find valuable. Moreover, she has managed to convey all this in a readable, practical, and easy-to-understand way.

Given that Helen Keller, perhaps the most famous American who was a deaf-blind person, was an integral part of the establishment and growth of the American Foundation for the Blind (AFB), we take a special pride in publishing a book that lies so close to the heart of two of her primary concerns—helping individuals with disabilities to realize their own potential and fostering understanding and communication among persons of all abilities and circumstances of life.

Carl R. Augusto
President and Executive Director
American Foundation for the Blind

PREFACE

The loss of both sight and hearing constitutes one of the severest disabilities known to human beings. Essentially, it deprives an individual of the two primary senses through which we acquire awareness of and information about the world around us, and it drastically limits effective communication and freedom of movement, which are necessary for full and active participation in society. Deaf-blindness creates greater dependence on others and unique problems of communication, mobility, and orientation that must be solved by using special methods and techniques.

During the last 50 years, much progress has been made in educating and training deaf-blind people to live more independently and in enabling them to overcome the acute sense of isolation and loneliness they often experience. New techniques and special aids and devices are helping to stretch horizons for deaf-blind people, and more trained professional workers are available to assist them with problems of adjustment and rehabilitation. But there has always been—and still is—a great need for relevant literature about deaf-blindness and how to minimize its problems.

When my friend Dona Sauerburger informed me that she was planning to publish a book on orientation and mobility for deaf-blind people, I was delighted. I knew that she was a highly qualified instructor who had the expertise and long-term experience with deaf-blind clients that would make such a book a major contribution to the literature of deaf-blindness. After reviewing the first rough copy, first from the viewpoint of a professional and then as a consumer, I knew that my original estimate had been confirmed.

Independence Without Sight or Sound is not merely a book about methods and techniques for teaching deaf-blind people. It is an integrated study of the needs of deaf-blind people who are reaching out to life and its human activities, written by an instructor who is understanding, sensitive, and dedicated to helping others. There are numerous examples from actual experience and discussions of practical applications, all presented with keen insight and held together by a clear awareness of the human factor.

If Dona Sauerburger's book had been available when I was a young man, it would have been invaluable to me as a consumer. It would have given me confidence to go out and meet the world, secure in the belief that I could rely on my knowledge and abilities, in spite of my disability of deaf-blindness. *Independence Without Sight or Sound* is a landmark contribution to the literature on deaf-blindness and human services.

Robert J. Smithdas
Assistant Director
Helen Keller National Center
for Deaf-Blind Youths and Adults

INTRODUCTION

*B*reathing in lilac and an April sun
I stand knee-deep in grass
my hand against a maple's tremulous song
as a west wind tiptoes through its young green leaves.

*S*oftly a feather falls upon my cheek
and I hold it in my hand,
wondering if a bird deep in the sky
has sent this silent note of spring to me
instead of the clear sweet silver ones I've lost?

*T*his is a soul's magnificence, that I
can touch this rhythm of the earth
and know for a little while that silence has voices
that vibrate from the muted heart of life:
and I will come away with a new patience,
and love to keep me safe against the dark!

—"Melody in April" in Smithdas, *Shared Beauty* (1982), p. 37.

We can never know what it is like to be both deaf and blind unless we are. I believe it is both more awesome and less awesome than we imagine. On the one hand, having limited access to what may seem to us to be inconsequential information—the facial expressions of those around us, fashions and fads, new products on the market, the daily goings-on of family members and co-workers, office and neighborhood gossip, incessant news reports—can be overwhelming and can leave an individual lonely even when surrounded by friends. On the other hand, people who are both deaf and blind often make full use of information from their other senses. We who can see or hear are frequently oblivious to our other senses because we normally get most of our information through our eyes or ears.

In his poem "Melody in April," Robert J. Smithdas (1982), who is deaf-blind, shares his impression of the rhythm of nature, which he enjoys through his remaining senses. If we neither saw nor heard, we could learn to notice the breeze that people stir when they open a door or walk by us. We could feel the vibrations of their footsteps on a wooden floor and know which way they are going and how fast they are trying to get there. The book that you are holding sometimes vibrates with the sounds around you; we could notice such effects in our surroundings and feel our whole body pound to the rhythm of music. We could feel the excitement or melancholy of our friends as they talk to us with their hands. Just as many people cannot imagine life without sight, many of us do not think of the wealth of information that is available through the senses of the blind person who cannot hear.

As Chapter 1 explains, most people who are considered deaf-blind are not totally blind and totally deaf. There is tremendous variety in the degrees of vision and hearing of deaf-blind persons, many different causes of vision and hearing loss, and a great range of individual abilities and needs among this group of people.

Some information about these issues is included in the chapters that follow. However, this book was written for those who know about visual impairments and their effect on people. Thus, it does not include fundamental information about such issues as low vision, adjustment to blindness, techniques of daily living, or orientation and mobility (O&M). The reader who is unfamiliar with the effects of the onset of visual or hearing disabilities should learn about them because these effects should be considered when planning any service. Nevertheless, it is important to remember that each person is an individual and that every generalization has its exceptions. For lay readers, some of the terms used in this book are explained in the Glossary.

Deaf-blind people usually have to find their way among agencies that serve blind people *or* deaf people because most communities do not offer comprehensive services to meet the unique needs of people who have both hearing and visual impairments. Often these agencies are reluctant or unprepared to serve this population, and deaf-blind people have to advocate for services and help the professionals learn how to work with them.

For example, Geraldine Lawhorn, who is deaf-blind, experienced typical difficulties when looking for an instructor. She said, "Not all teachers were willing to work with a deaf and blind student. Some declared themselves to be inadequate, others believed such a feat was impossible. . . . In a place of many peoples like New York, though [the right instructor was always found for me]. Always, the settlement was: 'I've never trained a deaf and blind person before, but I'll try.' That's all any teacher can do with any student—try" (Lawhorn, 1991, p. 83). In another example, I recently referred a deaf-blind client to a colleague whose competence I greatly respected and who I knew would be effective with the client. She responded, "I can't work with that client; I'm trained to work with people who are blind, not deaf-blind!"

I know how this colleague and other professionals feel when they consider working with a deaf-blind person. Twenty years ago, I protested emphatically when my supervisor asked me to interview a potential client who was deaf-blind. I reluctantly agreed to do it after my supervisor overrode my objection that I was not trained to teach

O&M to deaf-blind people. I had never even met a person who was deaf, much less a person who was deaf-blind, but I was told that the family could interpret for me.

When I arrived at the woman's home, I discovered that her husband and I could not understand each other because he was deaf, and her 12-year-old son said he could not communicate with her. As they watched, my mind raced, thinking of what to do with the pleasant-looking woman who was waiting expectantly.

I approached her, shook her hand, and decided to let her know why I was there by showing her the proper sighted guide technique. I placed her arm in the correct position and put her other hand on my head while I nodded yes. I then positioned her incorrectly and had her feel my head shake no. To illustrate the rationale for the proper technique, I guided her to the stairs on her porch. As I stepped down, I let her feel my arm drop and nodded yes. Then I positioned her too far forward and approached the stairs again, but this time indicated that she might fall.

Her face lit up with sudden understanding, and she used clear gestures to convey what she thought I had explained: "Never go outside alone; you will fall. Don't even go into your yard by yourself, or you may get hurt." Mortified by my failure, and not knowing what else to do, I bid everyone a hasty good-bye and fled to my car.

Luckily, this story had a happy ending. I later went back with an interpreter to see this woman. The client showed us how to print on her palm, which she said she preferred to sign language. With communication suddenly open to me, I proceeded to teach her everything that I normally teach blind clients. It was her delightful enthusiasm for learning, her sense of humor, and her determination to achieve independence that inspired me to learn sign language and to work with people who are deaf-blind.

I took several sign language classes, although because I had no contact with deaf people and only occasionally worked with deaf-blind clients, I forgot much of what I learned. However, my experiences with those clients were gratifying, and I sought every opportunity to work with them. In 1985 I became the community O&M instructor for Family Service Foundation's Institute on Deaf-Blindness in Lanham, Maryland. It was there, where I worked for three years, that my education really began.

I learned primarily from my deaf-blind clients, many of whom showed great courage in facing and overcoming a myriad of obstacles. One of the most gratifying aspects of my profession was to help them achieve a level of independence that some of them had not thought possible. The person who had the greatest influence on my work with deaf-blind people was Eleanor Macdonald, director of the institute. Her deep respect for clients, vast experience, creativity, and positive attitude were inspirational. I also learned about deaf culture from my co-workers, most of whom were deaf.

This book was written to help other service providers gain the insights and information that I needed when I began, so they can feel comfortable and be effective working with people who are deaf-blind. Such insights and information enabled my colleague to overcome her apprehension. She met with the client and they really hit it off, swiftly establishing effective communication. The services she provided were effective, and the experience was a positive one for both of them.

I hope that others will also consider working with deaf-blind people and have experiences as positive as that of one professional, whose eyes lit up when I mentioned deaf-blindness. He said that starting to work with a deaf-blind person was one of the scariest things he had ever done, but also one of the most rewarding. As Jack Wright, who is deaf-blind, commented: "I've known many intelligent workers who are afraid to meet deaf-blind people because they've never seen, met, or talked with one. If they would meet and get to know deaf-blind people, they'd learn a lot and become comfortable with them and influence other people. It is important for them to know that deaf-blind people are not helpless and can do well. They'd be very impressed if they could see what deaf-blind people can do. One thing I don't like is for them to pity deaf-blind people. We are very capable."

This book addresses issues, such as courtesies, interaction, assertiveness, and isolation, that are relevant for the many different types of professionals who work with deaf-blind people. Chapters in the later part of the book address topics that are of interest primarily to O&M specialists and deaf-blind travelers, although others may benefit from the information as well. The major part of the book addresses an issue that is a primary consideration when working with people who are deaf-blind: communication. Because clear, easy communication is so often taken for granted, many of us do not consider its importance. However, the frustration and misunderstandings that can occur and the inadequate services that are provided when communication is limited can be devastating, undermining even the best efforts of service providers. Because communication is so critical and must be considered when working with deaf-blind people, almost half the book is devoted to this subject.

Because I learned primarily through experiences—my own and those shared with me by others—this book includes numerous stories and examples. Many people contributed by reviewing the book and adding their ideas and experiences. Their comments and suggestions are included throughout the book. I am grateful to Stephen Ehrlich, who suggested the title for this book, and to the following reviewers:

People who are deaf-blind: Janice Adams, Maryland; Jeffrey Bohrman, Ohio; David Carrigan, Maryland; Chris Cook, California; Laura Engler, Maryland; Michelle Smithdas, New York; Robert J. Smithdas, New York; Caryn Spall, Florida; Dorothy Walt, Alaska; Boyd Wolfe, Arizona; and Jack Wright, Maryland.

Professionals with expertise in deaf-blindness: Paige Berry, deaf-blind consultant, Virginia Department for the Visually Handicapped, Richmond; Charlene R. Laba, coordinator, Adult and Continuing Education, Gallaudet University, Washington, DC; Leslie Leopold, program development specialist, Deaf-Blind Programs, College for Continuing Education, Gallaudet University; Monika McJannet-Werner, regional representative, Southeastern Region, Helen Keller National Center for Deaf-Blind Youths and

Adults, Atlanta, Georgia; Jeanne Prickett, coordinator of materials development, Deaf-Blind Project, American Foundation for the Blind, Washington, DC; Rustie Rothstein, regional representative, Southwestern Region, Helen Keller National Center for Deaf-Blind Youths and Adults, Van Nuys, California; Michelle Smithdas, instructor in communication, Helen Keller National Center for Deaf-Blind Youths and Adults, Sands Point, New York; Robert J. Smithdas, assistant director, Helen Keller National Center for Deaf-Blind Youths and Adults; Patricia M. Tesar, human development counselor, Gallaudet University; McCay Vernon, professor emeritus, Western Maryland College, Westminster and a psychologist in private practice; Dorothy Walt, rehabilitation counselor and coordinator, Deaf-Blind Affiliation Program, Alaska Center for Blind and Deaf Adults, Anchorage; Arlyce Watson, day program specialist, Institute on Deaf-Blindness, Family Service Foundation, Landover Hills, Maryland; and Julia Wright, hearing impaired resource teacher, Anne Arundel County Public Schools, Millersville, Maryland.

O&M specialists: Kathleen Deaver, O&M specialist, Sacramento County Office of Education, Sacramento, California; Elga Joffee, mobility instructor and national program associate, American Foundation for the Blind, New York; Doug McJannet, O&M specialist, Atlanta Public Schools, Georgia; Mary M. Michaud-Cooney, O&M specialist and deaf-blind consultant, Billerica, Massachusetts; Joani (Levy) Myers, O&M instructor, Prince Georges County Public Schools, Forrestville, Maryland; Cecelia Rose, O&M specialist, Columbia Lighthouse for the Blind, Washington, DC; Sandra Rosen, director, Programs in Orientation and Mobility, San Francisco State University, California; Barbara Seever, O&M specialist, Blind Focus, Kansas City, Missouri; William Van-Buskirk, O&M instructor and vision teacher, Frederick County Public Schools, Frederick, Maryland; Jenny Westman, O&M instructor, Virginia Department for the Visually Handicapped, Fairfax.

Other specialists: Robert Bayard and Jean Bayard, psychologists, Santa Clara, California; Diane Ignatius, assistant director of physical therapy, St. Jude Medical Center, Fullerton, California; Frederick Sauerburger, ophthalmologist, Waldorf, Maryland; Russell Williams, retired director, Blind Rehabilitation, Veterans Administration, Washington, DC; and Ted Zubrycki, trainer, Guiding Eyes for the Blind, Yorktown Heights, New York.

In addition, I would like to thank the following people for graciously allowing me to photograph them for this book (they are listed here in the order in which they appear): Chris Cook, Kathleen Deaver, Patricia Tesar, Caryn Spall, Jeanne Prickett, David Carrigan, Camille Morgan, John Foley, Lee Ivey, Jack Wright, Julia Wright, Kathy Lamon, Bernice Buck, and Arlyce Watson.

CHAPTER 1

COMMUNICATION

Clear communication is the indispensable ingredient for any successful interaction. When the communication is minimal, the benefits of the interaction are minimal. If you are an instructor, you need a high level of communication to teach the complex skills required for independent living and the efficient use of the remaining senses, explain the rationale behind techniques and when to use them, answer clients' questions, address their concerns, and discuss emotional issues. If you are a counselor or a consultant, good communication is just as critical.

Clear, full communication is necessary for any client. For deaf-blind clients, who often need accurate descriptions of what is occurring around them, it is even more important. Yet service providers often think that a minimal level of communication is acceptable with a deaf-blind person because they are not skilled in the person's language or method of communication. However, when they do not communicate fully, their interactions are fraught with frustration, their effectiveness is limited, and clients do not receive the services to which they are entitled.

DEAF-BLINDNESS: PRIMARY ISSUES

Most people who are considered deaf-blind are not totally blind and completely deaf. Although there are various definitions of deaf-blindness, the one used to define the population addressed in this book is a functional definition. That is, a person is deaf-blind if he or she has a combination of vision and hearing losses that together create a unique set of circumstances requiring adaptive techniques to function. Thus, a few of the people with whom I worked and about whom this book is written have profound or severe hearing losses and no useful vision. However, the majority are able to use their vision, their hearing, or both to some degree. Some have additional challenges, such as mental retardation; balance difficulties; physical disabilities requiring a walker, wheelchair, or cane; or impairments from strokes or diabetes.

The largest number of deaf-blind people are those who were born deaf and later lost their vision. Although a few lost their vision from unrelated causes, the most common cause of deaf-blindness among adults is Usher's syndrome, Types I and II. This hereditary syndrome incorporates a congenital hearing impairment with a loss of vision from retinitis pigmentosa (RP). RP is usually not noticed until late childhood or early adulthood, when a person has difficulty seeing at night and in dimly lit areas. Throughout the person's life, the visual field gradually decreases, usually leaving his or her central vision intact ("tunnel vision") until later in life. People with Usher's syndrome, Type I, are born with a severe to profound sensorineural hearing loss and, often, balance problems. The hearing loss in people with Usher's syndrome, Type II, can vary from mild to profound. Commonly, those with Type II function as hard-of-hearing people who use speech, rather than sign language (Duncan, Prickett, Finkelstein, Vernon, & Hollingsworth, 1988; Wynne, 1987).

Probably the second-largest group of people who are deaf-blind are those who were born with both visual and hearing impairments, at this time primarily as a result of the rubella epidemic of the 1960s, which caused neurological damage to the fetuses of women who contracted rubella. Other congenital visual and hearing impairments are the result of prenatal exposure to toxic substances and the complications of premature birth or birth trauma and range from mild to profound. Many, though not all, people with these congenital impairments are also developmentally delayed and have additional difficulties, including cardiac and respiratory problems and diabetes (Wynne, 1987).

Some people are born blind and lose their hearing later in life from the aging process, excessive environmental noise or a sudden loud noise, trauma to the head, medications or drugs, genetic diseases, high fever, diabetes, or kidney failure (Wynne, 1987). Others lose both their vision and their hearing later in life, sometimes years apart, from unrelated causes and sometimes simultaneously from a head injury, high fever or toxins, or a rare genetic syndrome. Some of the common causes of visual impairment are diabetic retinopathy, glaucoma, macular degeneration, and optic atrophy. Since vision and hearing are affected differently by each condition, you will need to learn about the specific visual and hearing characteristics of the person with whom you are working.

How a person becomes deaf-blind greatly affects his or her development and adjustment. A sudden and complete loss of vision or sight or both will have a different impact than will a loss that is gradual, fluctuating, or partial. Congenital deaf-blindness presents yet other ramifications. We continue to learn about the profound effects on the development of people's language when they are deaf before they learn how to speak and on the development of their posture and movement when they are blind before they learn to walk. Congenital blindness or deafness also has a profound impact on a person's learning and understanding of concepts about the world and everything in it. This impact is multiplied when the person is born with both a visual and a hearing impairment. For these reasons, it is important to be sensitive to the individual abilities and needs of deaf-blind people for effective communication to take place. Suggestions for interacting with someone who is deaf-blind are outlined in "Courtesies When Working with People Who Are Deaf-Blind" in this chapter.

TAKE YOUR TIME: GOOD COMMUNICATION IS ESSENTIAL

When you first meet a person who has a hearing and visual impairment, take the time to find out what methods of communication will be most comfortable and efficient for both of you (see Chapter 2). If you have difficulty establishing communication, those who know the person well or who referred him or her to you may have some suggestions.

There are no correct or incorrect methods of communication. There are only methods that allow the two of you to communicate as comfortably and efficiently as possible or methods that cause confusion, inconvenience, or frustration. Often, the most effective method is an interpreter. With people with minimal language or communication skills, be ready to heed and respond to all attempts at communication—gestures, vocal sounds, eye contact, body movements, and facial expressions.

As happens with all people, sometimes you and the deaf-blind person will misunderstand each other without being aware of it. When I was in charge of tours at a convention of the American Association of the Deaf-Blind, a deaf-blind man asked me about arrangements to tour Pike's Peak. I signed, "Call the train station and make reservations." He thought I meant that *I* would call the station. Fortunately, plenty of tickets were available when he arrived, and only later did we realize there had been a misunderstanding when he thanked me for making the reservations. Jeffrey Bohrman, who is deaf-blind, recalled that sometimes the instructor "would give me a set of instructions to follow, and we both seemed to understand each other. Then when the time came to use these instructions, I realized that I did not understand them."

Dorothy Walt, who is deaf-blind, suggests asking questions or giving each other feedback to determine if the message or information got through. If this reveals a misunderstanding or missing information, Jeff Bohrman says that rephrasing the message can often clarify it. Dorothy Walt also suggests that during the communication you allow time for rest or breaks so the person who is deaf-blind can "digest" what was learned.

Elga Joffee, mobility instructor and national program associate, American Foundation for the Blind (AFB), suggests that when one of you is not sure that the other person is getting the message, that person can repeat what he or she thinks the message was. For example, often when I spell words to clients, they repeat what I am spelling as

COURTESIES WHEN WORKING WITH PEOPLE WHO ARE DEAF-BLIND

The courtesies listed here were suggested by deaf-blind people and those who work with them (see also "Communicating with People whose Primary Language Is ASL" and "Establishing Roles" in this chapter).

Contact people who are deaf-blind on the hand, arm, or shoulder to avoid startling them. Use a light touch; a solid pat on the shoulder or back may be startling. Rather than tap them and then pull your hand away, leave your hand in contact with the person until he or she responds to you, to make it easier for the person to know where you are.

If you need to touch deaf-blind people somewhere besides the hand, arm or shoulder (for example, to point to something on their clothes or face) or to touch something they are holding, let them know what you are doing. One way to do this is to put your hand under theirs and then bring your hand toward them while their hand is on yours, so they realize your hand is approaching.

Identify yourself each time you initiate interaction. It is easier to identify yourself if you have a signal or name-sign that the deaf-blind person will recognize. Do not ask the person who is deaf-blind to try to guess who you are. It is patronizing, irritating, and rude. If the deaf-blind person recognizes you before you get a chance to identify yourself, do not demand that he or she repeat the performance the next time you meet.

Because you must usually stop what the deaf-blind person and you are doing in order to communicate that you are there, many people are reluctant to do so. Yet deaf-blind people are often disappointed that others do not announce themselves when they are near. Thus, if you frequently pass each other (for example as co-workers or neighbors), you might also make up a quick greeting signal (such as a light squeeze of the wrist) that allows you to identify yourself without interrupting either of you.

To guide people who are blind or deaf-blind, allow them to hold your arm as you walk. This technique allows them to remain in control while being guided, rather than being maneuvered by a guide who is holding their arm or pushing them.

Communicate directly with the deaf-blind person. If a deaf-blind person is accompanied by someone when you approach, address the deaf-blind person; do not direct your comments through the other person. Use a method of communication that the two of you can understand or ask if someone can interpret for you.

Let people who are deaf-blind know what is around them. When a deaf-blind person enters a room, describe the room and the people in it. When you leave, inform him or her that you will be gone. If you guide or drive the deaf-blind person to a destination, offer to describe the surroundings and the way he or she is facing before you leave, and, if needed for orientation or for balance, make sure he or she is in contact with furniture or a wall.

Be honest when you do not understand. When communicating with people who are deaf-blind, do not pretend to understand if you do not. Your honesty will be appreciated more than your attempt to be polite. Also, give the person opportunities to let you know when he or she is not sure what you meant, but do not ask repeatedly "Do you understand?"

Do not pull or push people who are deaf-blind. If the deaf-blind person is in someone's way or blocking a door, either ask that he or she move, or set up a signal (move the person's hand

(continued on next page)

in the direction in which you are requesting him or her to move, for instance) that informs the person that you want him or her to move.

Avoid communicating with the deaf-blind person when he or she is eating. Often the person will first have to clean his or her hands before putting his or her hand on yours to receive your message. If you need to tell the person something, you might print the message succinctly with your finger (letters about 3 inches high) on the person's upper arm or back.

Avoid placing the deaf-blind person's hand on objects. Instead, when you help people who are deaf-blind find a stair railing, the back of a chair, or a door handle, for example, tell them you are putting your hand on the object while their hand is on yours. Then they can find the object by sliding their hand off yours as you remove your hand. Do not push the person's hand onto the object because it is awkward and may be painful if the object is sharp or rough or if the deaf-blind person's hand is sore from a cut or bruise.

When people with restricted visual fields are watching you, do not move quickly to the side. If they are trying to follow you or look at your signs and you move too quickly to the side, they may lose you. If they cannot find you, you might let them know where you are by touching one of their arms or hands.

For appointments at the deaf-blind person's home, find out how he or she will know you have arrived. Be sure to be prompt—often the person leaves the door unlocked, is waiting outside, or checks frequently to see if you are there. To announce your arrival, you might approach with heavy steps so the person can feel the floor vibrate.

Do not misconstrue the deaf-blind person's normal speaking voice as a display of strong emotion. Some people conclude from the unusual voice inflections or the emphatic signs and facial expressions with which many people who are deaf and deaf-blind communicate that they are agitated or perturbed. It is important to realize that the voice may be the person's normal speaking voice, and that eloquence in sign language usually involves dynamic, intense expression.

I go (sometimes anticipating the rest of the sentence, which saves time if they are right). If you are not sure what the other person is signing or voicing, repeat it back in whatever method of communication he or she understands.

Most people feel frustrated and patronized when others pretend that they understand. Deaf people frequently complain that when hearing people do not understand a deaf person, they often pretend that they do. If you think you do not grasp something that the deaf-blind person says, let him or her know. When I tell people that I am unable to understand them even after repeated efforts, they may decide it is not worth explaining or try again under different circumstances (such as with an interpreter or when they can show me what they are explaining). Your honesty will be appreciated more than your attempts to be polite. (Additional principles and suggestions relating to working with deaf-blind persons are outlined in "Philosophy of Teaching People Who Are Deaf-Blind.")

Many people who are deaf also pretend to understand when they do not. For exam-

PHILOSOPHY OF TEACHING PEOPLE WHO ARE DEAF-BLIND

- The effective worker helps each client achieve his or her own level of autonomy and ignores clichés and generalizations about the potential ability of people who are deaf-blind. Some generalizations are easy to recognize as erroneous, such as that people who are deaf-blind cannot learn to use a cane because its use requires the sense of hearing and that children who are deaf-blind cannot use braille because the manual alphabet does not include the braille contractions. Other clichés, such as that few deaf-blind persons will travel independently, may not be so apparently false, but I have found them equally untrue.

  Perhaps the reason that generalizations are usually false is that they do not take individuals into account. Dorothy Walt, who coordinates a program for deaf-blind people and is herself deaf-blind, commented, "It is important for people working with the client who is deaf-blind to look at the person first and the disability last. Many people tend to look at the disability first and the possible limitations (rightly or wrongly imagined), which may interfere with their perception of the individual's personality and capabilities."
- The only person who should make decisions for an individual who is deaf-blind is that deaf-blind individual. The instructor's role is to empower the client to make decisions by helping him or her to gather the necessary information, understand the consequences of the decisions, and develop the skills and techniques needed to achieve his or her own goals (see Chapter 6).
- One definition of independence is freedom from the influence, guidance, or control of others. Although people who are deaf-blind may need the assistance of others to do certain things, they should decide when and where they need the assistance and arrange for it. The instructor resists the opportunity to step in and take over and gives the person the opportunity to act independently, to increase the person's self-reliance, self-confidence, and pride (see "When the Instructor Should Step In" in Chapter 4).
- The effective instructor is flexible and creative. If the client prefers a technique that is novel or unorthodox but safe, there is no reason he or she should not use it. The instructor keeps in mind the principles and rationales behind the techniques being taught and adapts them to suit each individual's needs.

ple, when he first lost a significant amount of his hearing and vision, one man who had difficulty understanding others said that when people asked if he understood them, "not wanting to inconvenience them I often replied affirmatively. Often they would make me repeat what they said to me, and I found this to be more frustrating."

This "silent misunderstanding" could be disastrous. As the man explained, "when I lost my job, I found out later that I did not 'hear' the interpreters telling me the facts. Yet I know that they explained them because I did remember understanding some of the words used in that part of the conversation." Try to make the deaf-blind person feel comfortable enough to be honest and tell you when he or she does not comprehend what you are saying by being patient when messages need to be repeated or reworded or by offering to try alternative methods of communication that may be more effective.

People who are learning how to communicate again after a loss of vision or hearing, have few opportunities to interact, or are using a new method of communication may need to proceed slowly. I repeatedly have found out the hard way that it does no good to try to speed things up. When I try to communicate more quickly, the other person usually becomes frustrated and feels inadequate, sometimes to the point of feeling hopeless or preferring to withdraw from interactions with others. I often feel the same way when others insist on communicating too fast for me.

To avoid having to communicate too fast, I allow plenty of time for the interaction, sometimes by scheduling three hours for lessons that would normally require one hour or by planning lessons that cover less material in the given time. Usually I feel pressured to communicate too fast when choices have to be made quickly (such as when we arrive at the front of a cafeteria line) or when I try to interpret for others who want to go too fast (for example, when people approach us in public or when I accompany someone to a physician's office). As much as possible, plan ahead so you can give information about choices beforehand and avoid situations in which communication must be provided immediately. The person who communicates slowly may need to prepare others to expect slow communication and arrange more time than usual for appointments and meetings.

You may find that some people tend to dominate the conversation. When people have difficulty understanding, they can comprehend better if they know the topic of conversation and if the other person does not communicate more than short answers. They can arrange to do this if they initiate the topic of conversation and control where the discussion leads. If a deaf-blind person is doing so, try to make it easier for him or her to understand you by changing communication methods, getting an interpreter, or slowing down.

It is easy to notice the tendency for others to dominate a conversation when we are communicating using a method with which we are comfortable and with which the other person is at a disadvantage, such as when we use spoken English with a person who is hard-of-hearing. However, many of us also try to dominate the conversation when we communicate using a method, such as sign language, in which our skills are limited and we are at a disadvantage. Watch for your tendency to do this, and do not discourage your client from bringing up topics of concern or responding fully to you. If you have difficulty understanding or if either of you are getting frustrated enough that you are holding back from communicating, get an interpreter.

COMMUNICATION WITH SIGN LANGUAGE

American Sign Language

American Sign Language (ASL) has evolved naturally as a language among deaf people in the United States and Canada the same way that spoken languages have. As a language with its own syntax and rules for grammar, it is *not* a representation of English on the hands. Just as English has been enriched by borrowing from other languages, ASL has borrowed and incorporated terms and concepts from spoken English (although this does not mean that it has become English). It also has incorporated many French signs that were brought to the United States in 1816 by Laurent Clerc, a deaf man whom Thomas Hopkins Gallaudet recruited to teach American deaf students. For that reason, ASL has more in common with French Sign Language than with British Sign Language.

Because ASL is structurally different from English, when it is transliterated (translated word for word) into English, it sounds bizarre, just as any language would. The Spanish phrase *antes de irme para Mexico* sounds strange when transliterated as "before of to go me for Mexico." The ASL phrase that means, "Did you go to Mexico?" is literally, "Touch finish Mexico you?" When deaf people who are verbal in ASL but not in English try to write or understand English (which for them is a second language), some people mistakenly think they have minimal language skills. However, this assumption is similar to the assumption that a scientist who speaks only Spanish has minimal language skills.

Today there is a lot of confusion about ASL. Many people with whom I spoke still think that ASL is a version of English. One teacher of deaf children told me that she is starting to use ASL; by this she meant that she is saying English while signing only the important words (omitting such words as *the* and *to*). Signed words in English order, even if some words are dropped, is no more ASL than Spanish words used with English syntax would be considered Spanish. What this teacher (and many people who believe they are learning "sign language") is using is either Signed English or Pidgin Signed English.

Signed English was made up in the early 1970s by educators who wanted to use signs in the classroom to help teach deaf children English (Hoemann, 1976; Markowicz, 1977). It is a codified system of arbitrary signs and symbols representing English words. Names for other codified sign systems are Signed Exact English, Siglish, and Exact English. Since there are no specific ASL signs for many English words and suffixes (just as there are no English words for many ASL signs), numerous signs had to be invented or adapted from ASL signs. Each of these made-up signs, as well as signs borrowed from ASL, represents an English word, and the words are used in the order that the words are spoken in English. Even though many of the signs used in Signed English are the same as those used in ASL, this system is not the same as the natural sign language developed in the deaf community.

Pidgin Signed English (PSE) is a combination of Signed English and ASL and can be anything from almost "pure" ASL to almost Exact Signed English. Hearing people who are just beginning to learn ASL often sign more in English than in ASL; as they become more experienced, their PSE better approximates ASL. Many deaf people who use mainly ASL will use PSE or even Signed English to communicate with people who do not know ASL.

Many people who use PSE make their signs while thinking in English (or even speaking English) but, like the teacher mentioned earlier, do not interpret words that have no sign in ASL (such as *the* and *a*). Likewise, they often do not sign plurals, pronouns, or the tense of the verbs, since there are no specific ASL signs for them. Thus they may interpret such sentences as "Did you go there?" and "Go there" with exactly the same signs. The listener can usually tell the difference from the context in which the sentence was signed, from the person's facial expression (a quizzical look for a question and an assertive look for an imperative), and sometimes by reading lips.

Some deaf people who understood PSE when they were sighted find it hard to understand it when they become blind and need to follow the signs tactilely because they can no longer read lips and watch facial expressions. They may understand ASL better, although, since facial expression is also an important part of ASL, the information conveyed by facial expressions would have to be conveyed by the hands. For example, a quizzical facial expression can be replaced by the quizzical gesture of turning the hands palm up or by the sign for *question.* Others would understand PSE better if more of the English was translated into signs. For example, to say "Did you go there?" it may be helpful to include the sign that indicates past action or to fingerspell *did* and to add the sign for question at the end. (In fingerspelling, each letter is expressed by different shapes of the hand. See Chapter 2 for more information.)

Attitudes toward Sign Languages

Until the 1960s most people did not realize that deaf people had a language of their own (Baker & Battison, 1980). Many thought that deaf people were just using glorified gestures or drawing pictures or icons in the air and doubted that deaf people could convey complicated conceptual meanings (see experimenters' concerns in Appendix B). These misconceptions are still prevalent even among educators of deaf children (Cokely, 1980, p. 153).

Today, linguists maintain that all languages "are equally complex and capable of expressing any idea. A language which appears to be simple in some respects is likely to be more complex in others" (Markowicz, 1977, p. 15). However, for many years ASL was not considered a language. Deaf children who were caught signing to each other at school were punished (sometimes with a ruler rapped on the hands), and many deaf people were embarrassed to be seen using sign language.

In the 1960s, linguistic research by William C. Stokoe, Jr., and others determined that the sign languages of deaf people, including ASL, are indeed authentic languages, as complex and sophisticated as any others. Partly because of this recognition, many schools now use signs to help communicate with deaf students (Stevens, 1980), although they may not recognize the value of ASL as a language or incorporate the language into their "total communication" system (Cokely, 1980; Erting, 1980).

When Stokoe published his research, many deaf people did not consider their sign language to be worthy of such scientific investigation or to be culturally equal to a spoken language. They now have an increasing sense of power and significance and are recognizing and asserting their right to use their own language. Trybus (1980, p. 215) wrote that "deaf clients are likely to increasingly demand that practitioners substantially improve their understanding of the culture of deafness and their Sign Language ability as an emblem of that understanding. . . . These practitioners, in turn, can be expected to respond with resentment, confusion, and some bitterness, when their attempts to be of service are rebuffed or criticized by their actual or potential clients." Nevertheless, many service providers today understand and support the right of deaf people to have access to communication through their own language, ASL.

People Who Use ASL

It is important to repeat that for some people who are deaf or deaf-blind, English is a second language that they do not understand as well as their native language, ASL—even if you convey the English in a modality that they can perceive, such as fingerspelling or written notes, or by using encoded English, such as Signed English or PSE. How can a person understand each word in an English sentence and yet not understand the sentence? To illustrate, see if you can understand the following ASL sentences, each word of which has been translated (from Humphries, Padden, & O'Rourke, 1980, p. 253, 146, 112):

1. Test yourself worry you?
2. That-one you good-friend my brother you?
3. Friend I see none since.

If you are not familiar with ASL, even though you understand each word, the meanings of the foregoing sentences probably are not clear. If you saw these statements signed during a conversation, you might try to guess what the sentences mean and let the speaker continue in the hope that you could get the gist of the meaning from the context.

It is the same with people who use ASL but do not understand English well. They may understand the meaning of each English word and of most sentences, but may not fully understand or may misunderstand some of the sentences that you may sign, write, or fingerspell in English. If you are not skilled in the use of ASL and do not have a competent interpreter, ASL users and you will not understand each other, and the result will be frustration for both of you and slower progress in the provision of services.

Just for fun, see if you understood the ASL sentences just listed. The following are the correct translations:

1. Are you worried about the test?
2. Are you the one that's a good friend of my brother?
3. I haven't seen my friend for a long time.

If you plan to learn sign language and want to communicate better with people who do not fully understand English (or PSE), it will be more beneficial to take courses in ASL than in Signed English. If you are teaching a deaf child, however, the school may require that you use Signed English because it is assumed that it will improve the child's comprehension of English (although this supposition has been questioned; see, for example, Cokely, 1980). I found that after learning ASL signs, it was easy to learn the adaptations and invented signs needed for Signed English.

Who Uses Which Kind of Communication?

Each person's background helps determine whether he or she uses ASL, English, or other systems of communication. For example, according to Woodward (1980), people whose parents were deaf or who learned signs before age 6 tend to sign with a syntax that is more purely ASL than those whose parents were not deaf or who learned signs later in life.

Although I refer to ASL and English here, the main points also apply to people in other countries that have a native sign language. For example, deaf people in France may prefer either French Sign Language or the French language. If they prefer the latter, they may use signs that follow the word order of the French spoken language, rather than French Sign Language, just as Signed English follows the order of spoken English. Likewise in England, they would use either British Sign Language or English.

Some people who are deaf or deaf-blind do not use any standard language or system of communication. They may never have been exposed to a language in a modality that they can perceive and use. Perhaps they were raised in a home or institution in which the family or staff made up their own communication system. Or they may have cognitive impairments that interfere with their ability to process the abstract information of language.

On the basis of their background, most people who are deaf or deaf-blind belong to one of the following categories of communicators:

- Congenitally deaf people whose native language is ASL. For these people, English is a second language that they may or may not understand well. If they lose their vision, they usually prefer to continue using ASL (tactilely).
- Congenitally deaf people who were raised using the "oral method" of communication. English is the native language of these people and thus they prefer to speak English and read lips. Some have also learned ASL (or more often PSE), but English is their primary language.

  If they become blind, some may use signs, but others prefer spelled-out English (such as fingerspelling or braille) as their primary method of communication. Since sign language depends on visual-spatial concepts and is more difficult to learn without vision, some people who are losing their sight learn how to sign while they still can see.

- People who learned English before they lost their hearing. These people usually can continue to speak English and prefer a mode of receptive communication that is based on English, such as a combination of PSE, lipreading (if they have enough vision), assistive listening devices, or written notes. Some people become proficient in ASL, but many do not. If they are blind, a few may prefer tactile ASL, but most prefer signs in syntax that is more like English (PSE) or spelled-out English, such as fingerspelling, braille, or occasionally printing letters on their palm.
- People who can hear well enough to understand spoken English. Some of these people prefer to use signs to augment their listening and their speech, but others rely solely on spoken English.
- People who have "minimal language skills," which means that they lack competence in ASL, English, or any standard language. Such people may have congenital multiple impairments or have been isolated and hence were unable to learn a language or had no opportunity to do so. They may use a system of "home signs" (made-up signs) and natural gestures or symbols, such as object cues (objects that symbolize an object or concept).
- People who have "minimal communication skills." These people are not able to use any system of communication, perhaps because they could not or had no opportunity to learn a communication system. They may use gestures, vocal sounds, body movements, and facial expressions to communicate, or they may not respond or interact to any extent.

When Is an Interpreter Necessary?

Some service providers believe that the obvious solution to communicating with people who are deaf-blind is to learn their language or method of communication. Dinsmore (1959, p.8) wrote, "When a worker undertakes to serve a deaf-blind person, it is his responsibility to establish communication in order to have [a] direct relationship, rather than working through an interpreter. If the client uses a given method of communication, the worker should learn that method." I subscribed to this philosophy and taught the best I could without an interpreter, even before I could sign well. As mobility instructor Cecelia Rose noted, "I did not realize that an interpreter was an option for me. I felt obligated to improve my signs in preparation for working with my deaf-blind client."

It would be ideal if the worker became skilled in the client's language and method of communication. This may be possible if the client understands English well and can use a method that the worker already knows or can learn quickly, such as print on palm, fingerspelling, lipreading, written notes, braille, or Teletouch (see Chapter 2 for more information about these methods of communication). However, it is impractical for those who work only occasionally with deaf-blind people to invest the time and effort needed to become proficient in sign language. Those who have few opportunities to use the language soon forget what they learned. It is also important to remember that some deaf people understand only ASL, not English or even Signed English.

Theresa Smith, a nationally respected interpreter with many years' experience working with people who are deaf-blind, wrote (personal communication, 1991), "It has been my consistent experience that while the communication often seems adequate to the Hearing person, the Deaf or Deaf-Blind person is being polite at the expense of really understanding. When this happens, Deaf and Deaf-Blind people may modify their own questions (such as asking only yes-no questions) and avoid making meaningful comments, because they know that the Hearing person probably will not be able to understand or communicate such substantial information. At best, they are putting mental energy into just getting the language—energy which would be better spent on actually thinking about the valuable ideas the instructor is giving them."

The inability of a deaf person to understand English has little to do with intelligence, as does the inability of any person to become fluent in a second language. Some deaf users of ASL who have a poor understanding of English are college graduates or are successfully working at administrative jobs in organizations where co-workers understand sign language.

For example, one evening an intelligent woman who is deaf-blind and I were using our TDDs (telecommunication devices for the deaf) to type to each other over the phone (see "Communication Devices" in Chapter 2). We could normally communicate well when using signs. I wanted to include her in the survey reported later in this section and asked her if she would want an interpreter if her mobility instructor could not sign. I tried three different ways to phrase the question, but I could not get the point across. We finally agreed to discuss it in person when I could sign. She understood my first explanation in sign. It is not surprising that she is one of those who would prefer to use an interpreter.

Another woman who was raising her family and had a good job in data entry was congenitally deaf and losing her vision. During our interview, I recommended a book that would be helpful to her. I also told her that if she learned braille, she could continue to read the television telecaptions (using a new invention that transforms them into braille) after she lost her vision. She explained, however, that even now, when she can see, she does not understand telecaptions or books well because of her limited grasp of English.

Some people are not as candid. They may nod in agreement or feign understanding, and you may mistakenly think that they understand English (or Signed English or PSE) well. Conversely, some deaf people who understand English well believe that because they are deaf, they can never fully master English (Trybus, 1980, p. 213) and are reluctant to be in situations that require good English skills.

I asked nine people whether they would prefer an interpreter or would want their instructor to use a method of direct communication (such as notes or fingerspelling) if their mobility instructor was not proficient with signs or ASL. All were congenitally deaf and adventitiously visually impaired except one, who lost both vision and hearing in adulthood; all but two had useful remaining vision. Seven (including the adventitiously deaf person and both people with no useful vision) would prefer an interpreter and two would prefer to communicate with the instructor without an interpreter. One of the two, who relies primarily on lipreading, preferred a "one-on-one" relationship with the instructor and thought that "a third person would be a nuisance." The other person, who primarily uses ASL, said she relies on observation and thought it would be difficult to watch the interpreter while trying to observe the technique because her visual field is severely restricted. When I explained that mobility instruction does not consist only of demonstration, she said it would be good to have an interpreter for the first and last lessons, when she thought it would be important to be able to communicate.

The seven who would want an interpreter included four whose primary language was ASL. They said they would want an interpreter because "I'm lousy at writing" and "I don't understand writing well—I wouldn't understand everything." The primary language of the other three was English. One was a young woman who used PSE. She explained, "If I could still see well, I could deal with the communication problem, but being blind now, too, it would be too frustrating to work without an interpreter if the instructor doesn't know how to sign." The second person, who did not learn to sign until he started to lose his vision, agreed. The third person, who had lost his vision and hearing as an adult, preferred to use ASL.

Thus, if you cannot competently use a communication method that the deaf-blind person can fully understand, ask if he or she would prefer an interpreter. Be sure to explain whether your interaction will involve just the demonstration and learning of techniques or will sometimes require in-depth communication. Discourage polite answers.

Because clear, comfortable communication is essential, you should be flexible about changing the arrangements when necessary. If the person decides to use an interpreter or communicate without one and it does not work out, try other alternatives until communication is satisfactory.

Communicating with People Whose Primary Language Is ASL

If you do not know ASL well and the person does not know English well, an interpreter will be necessary (see "Direct Communication through an Interpreter" later in this chapter). The following points may be useful when you are communicating with a person whose primary language is ASL. They may also enable you to anticipate some of the misunderstandings that may occur when the ASL user and the public communicate with each other.

Get to the Point

In our hearing culture, people often begin with introductory information and gradually build up to their main points. For example, speakers may warm up with a few jokes, then perhaps give some anecdotes or facts that will eventually lead to the point they are making.

Several interpreters have told me that these introductory remarks are difficult to translate because ASL users usually do the opposite: They begin with their main point or points and then fill in with details and information. This progression would seem to be beneficial for teaching or working with any person, since the points may be better understood and retained. (If I were following this recommendation, the next sentence would have been my first, instead of my last in this section). You should begin with the point you are trying to make, followed by your explanations and general supporting data.

Set the Stage

It helps to set the stage by presenting the global picture first, then the details. For example, before beginning to orient a deaf-blind person to a room, first explain that you are going to describe the room. Start with the general features of the room, such as its shape, size, and where the person is standing, before explaining the furnishings and other details.

Follow the Order of Events

ASL follows the sequence in which the events occurred or will occur. As a corollary, Paige Berry, a consultant on deaf-blindness, added that the cause of an action is usually named first, then its effect. For example, when I told a deaf-blind man that my friend was a retired painter, I signed in PSE, "<friend> <is> <retire> <painter>." The man assumed that my friend retired then started painting. I should have signed, "<friend> <in-the-past> <work> <paint> <finish> <retire>." In English, I could have said, "My friend was a painter and then retired."

This difference between ASL and English may cause problems when a person who understands only ASL communicates with the English-speaking public (see "Public Responses" in Chapter 3). If you write, "Turn left when you get to the corner," the person may turn left, then walk to the corner. It is clearer to say, "Go to the corner and turn left." In this situation, for example, the person who is deaf-blind may give a note saying,

> Please write directions to the drug store for me. I am deaf and can't see well. Thank you.
>
> First ____________________
>
> Then ____________________
>
> Next ____________________
>
> Next ____________________

Technical Terms

Do not dwell on technical terms in English. For example, it was difficult for one mobility instructor to convey the concept of the three-point touch technique (see Glossary) through the interpreter. It may have been easier first to demonstrate the technique to the interpreter, who could then describe it, or to use pictorial descriptions (see "'Pictorial Description'" in Chapter 2).

Idioms and Metaphors

Most languages have idioms and metaphors that, if taken literally, make no sense to outsiders. In ASL "<train> <zoom-away>!" can mean you missed the point and it is too late to go over it again (similar to "you've missed the boat").

It is easy to forget that we use idioms and metaphors—they are such an important part of any culture, yet they can be confusing to people, including ASL users, for whom English is a second language because they often take the words literally or misunderstand the expressions. After a grueling lesson one day, I told a college student who is deaf and visually impaired that she is a "good sport." We had walked through a blizzard—using her cane to find the sidewalk under 18 inches of snow, huddled together laughing and freezing—and I admired her spunk. She thought I meant she was good at sports and told me she had skied several times.

Negatives

Arlyce Watson, a deaf supervisor of a program for people who are deaf-blind, said that double negatives can be confusing because they are not used in ASL. (They are confusing to English speakers as well.) Examples of troublemakers are "not unless," "not without," and "not only that, but." It is also confusing to use negative adjectives with another negative, such as "not ineligible" and "never invalid."

Also avoid questions with a negative ("You aren't going to the store, are you?"). This English convention can be confusing to native speakers of other languages, including ASL, because it is not clear what a yes or a no answer means. "Aren't you [are you not] going to the store?" could be answered, "Yes, I am not going to the store."

Learning the "Correct" Sign

Regardless of how proficient one becomes in sign language, there is always room for improvement. There is no need to argue which sign is "correct"—the one described in a textbook and classroom or the one that a specific deaf-blind person prefers. Like any natural language that has developed different dialects, people in different geographic areas have their own signs for many things. Even within a given area, there may be more than one sign for the same concept. In Maryland, some signs are used only by recent graduates of Gallaudet University; others are used by deaf people in the metropolitan Washington, DC, area; and still others are used by deaf people in Baltimore. Sometimes, when I learn a new sign from one person, the next person does not recognize it. Therefore, be flexible, learn as much as you can, and be prepared to try something else if the deaf-blind person does not understand you. When he or she uses a sign that you do not recognize, do not be embarrassed to ask what it means and to learn from him or her.

When working with some deaf people as well as with a hearing client for whom I used a Spanish-language interpreter, I noticed that the learners felt proud when they could teach the teacher. If I made a mistake or expressed something awkwardly, some clients gladly showed me how to do it better. Rather than feel indignant about the correction, I considered it an opportunity not only to learn more of their language, but to allow them to feel a sense of accomplishment at a time when they had to learn so much to regain control over their lives.

However, you should not take advantage of the time that you are supposed to be providing service to learn another language. Some clients will be exasperated with professionals who plan to work without an interpreter so that they, the professionals, can learn.

DIRECT COMMUNICATION THROUGH AN INTERPRETER

If you have watched the president of the United States talking with foreign dignitaries, you have an idea of how interpreters are used. The president does not look at the interpreter and say, "Tell your leader that we want to expand trade between our countries." He looks directly at the dignitary and speaks to him or her, while the interpreter unobtrusively translates what he has said. The president would never think to turn to the interpreter and ask his or her opinion on how to expand trade. The interpreter would probably be fired immediately if he or she stopped to offer the president or the dignitary advice about such issues as trade between the countries.

Speak directly to the person who is hearing impaired, not to the interpreter, and do not expect the interpreter to answer questions or get involved in the conversation (see Figure 1). You are there to provide a service to the client, and the interpreter is there to facilitate the communication. If either you or the client involve the interpreter in the conversation, it may diminish the direct relationship between you and the client.

Even if it were ethical for the interpreter to be involved, it is often difficult for a competent interpreter to do so. If you have ever tried to type a paper from an audiotape or manuscript or transcribe text into braille, or vice versa, quickly and efficiently, you probably were not always aware of what you were typing or transcribing. In the same manner, the interpreter often is not aware of the content of the message, but is processing the message to translate it into the other person's language or code. It is usually too much to expect an interpreter to do an efficient, professional job of interpreting and to be involved in the conversation or to remember details about it afterward.

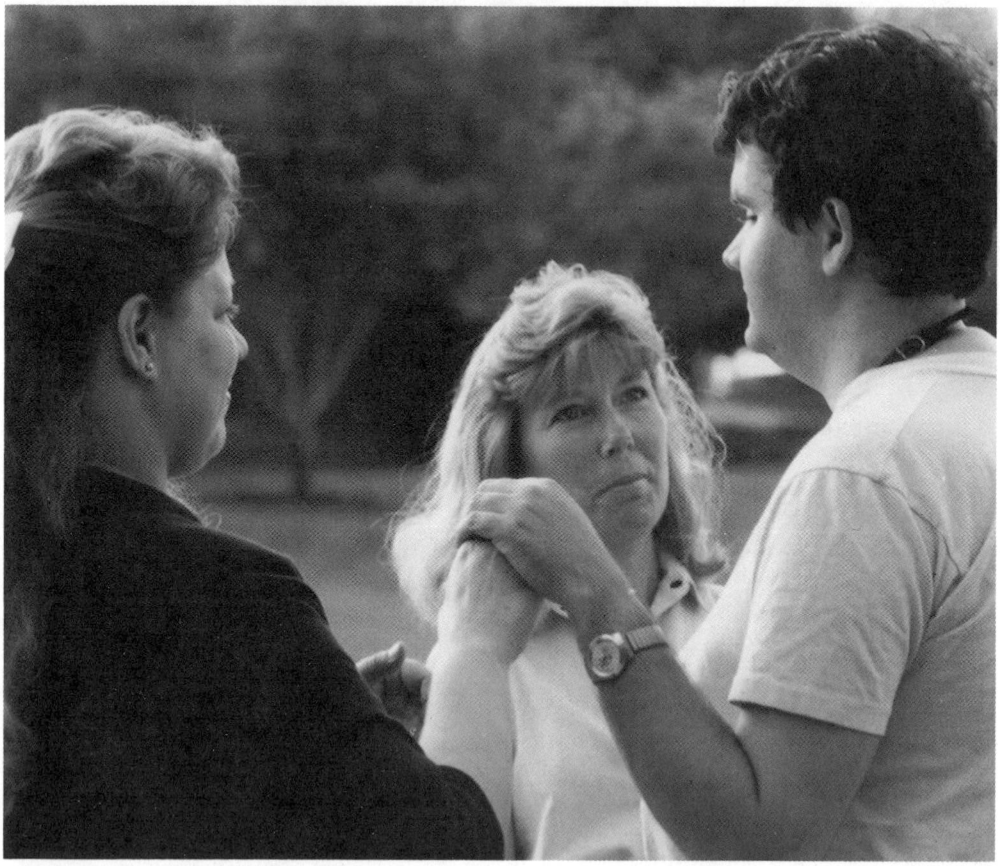

Figure 1. Speak directly to the person who is hearing impaired. In this situation, the instructor (*middle*) speaks to her client, a deaf-blind young man, rather than to the interpreter. The interpreter (*left*) is fingerspelling what the instructor is saying.

The interpreter cannot translate word by word or even phrase by phrase into another language, such as ASL. Because the syntax is different, the interpreter must comprehend the sentence or the whole concept before translating it. For example, I once watched an interpreter translate for a speaker at a conference. The speaker paused between phrases, and the interpreter was never sure when to proceed. At one point the speaker said, "We contacted our congressmen—and they listened." She paused as if finished, so the interpreter translated. However, the speaker then added "for once!" This meant that in the past, the congressmen did **not** listen. Because the concepts in ASL are conveyed in the order in which they happen, the interpreter had to start all over again. He signed that she contacted the congressmen, they did not listen—and finally they listened.

In addition, some words in English have more than one meaning. Thus, even if the interpreter is translating into Signed English, he or she will sometimes need to hear the whole sentence to get the context. I once interpreted while a stranger talked to my client and me during a lesson. He waited for me to interpret each phrase before continuing. On departing, he said, "I must go now—because I have patience." I thought this statement was a bit odd, but I interpreted it. The man then went on to say, "waiting for me at the hospital."

Establishing Roles

The interaction will progress more smoothly if every person's role is clarified. The deaf-blind person and you should determine how the interpreter can best be utilized. Ideally, the interpreter remains impartial, but in reality some people who have a special relationship with the interpreter prefer that the interpreter is involved in the conversation. When this is the case, the interpreter should still translate everything that is communicated. As was already explained, this can be difficult for the interpreter, and if it does not work out smoothly, the roles may need to be redefined.

When it is decided that the interpreter will remain impartial, if you want to say something to the interpreter, you should ask the deaf-blind person if the interpreter can step out of the role and communicate directly with you. This courtesy allows the deaf-blind person to determine the interpreter's role and to understand why the interpreter and you are communicating without directly involving him or her. Of course the deaf-blind person should extend the same courtesy to you if he or she wants to communicate directly to the interpreter.

Many interpreters are not accustomed to interpreting for people who are deaf-blind. It is important for them to remember that the person is visually impaired, so that while they interpret, they must let him or her know who is speaking. They also need to convey the speaker's expression (is the speaker smiling or frowning in response to the deaf-blind person? Is he or she leaning forward with attention or looking at some papers?), as well as any visual or auditory clues about the context of the communication (does the speaker seem to be distracted by traffic conditions; a radio, television, or ringing phone; or other people making jokes or trying to get the speaker's attention?).

For some reason, people are sometimes reluctant to communicate with deaf or deaf-blind people, even through an interpreter. Instead they speak to the interpreter or try to involve the interpreter in the conversation. When they do, the interpreter should stay impartial and translate accurately, so the deaf person realizes what is happening and knows who is saying what to whom. It is then the deaf person's responsibility to correct the situation by explaining the interpreter's role or by allowing the interpreter to step out of that role and respond to the other person and the interpreter's responsibility to translate the explanation.

Some people who are deaf or deaf-blind do not have much experience using an interpreter, other than friends or family members who interject or make decisions for them (sometimes without translating fully). Thus, they are not familiar with the professional interpreter's proper role or code of ethics. Mobility instructor Jenny Westman noticed that if someone spoke to the interpreter, rather than to her deaf-blind clients, the clients sometimes relied on the interpreter to answer for them. If a goal of your program is to help clients become experienced and confident enough to make their own decisions, they may have to learn how to use an interpreter properly (see "Interpreting for the Public" in Chapter 3).

It is not the interpreter's role to let the parties know when one seems to be misunderstanding the other, so you and the deaf-blind person need to be alert for indications that the other person may not understand (see "Take Your Time: Good Communication Is Essential" in this chapter). When a misunderstanding occurs, it is not the interpreter who rephrases the message or tries to explain it more clearly, but the person who first tried to convey it. The interpreter then translates the second message. If you did not understand the deaf-blind person (as translated by the interpreter), ask the deaf-blind person, not the interpreter, for clarification.

The role of interpreters for people who are deaf-blind includes guiding them and describing the environment for them (*Strategies for Serving Deaf-Blind Clients*, 1984). When an interpreter is used during orientation and mobility (O&M) lessons, there may be a conflict of roles because the mobility instructor also usually guides clients and describes the environment. Therefore, it may be wise to discuss beforehand what each of you will do. For example, the instructor could guide the client, as a way of establishing rapport and helping the client to get to know the instructor.

If the objective of the lesson is to have the client determine what is in the environment or orient himself or herself, the interpreter's independent description may defeat the purpose. In addition, sometimes the instructor does not want certain information conveyed. For example, when instructor Kathy Deaver used an interpreter while assessing a client's vision, she asked the client if he could scan and see a certain object. Like many verbs that are directional in sign language, the sign for "look at" normally involves moving the hand toward the object. Thus, in translating the request, the interpreter gestured toward the object, so Kathy was unable to learn if the client could have found it himself.

To avoid these problems, mobility instructor and AFB national program associate Elga Joffee suggests that before the lesson you explain to the interpreter what you want to say and what you do not want conveyed, so the translation will impart exactly what you intend. If an unforeseen situation during the lesson necessitates more consultation with the interpreter, obtain the client's consent to stop and explain it to the interpreter.

Joffee also points out that for sessions during which you must monitor the client's safety (such as mobility or cooking lessons), it is important to specify everyone's role for situations when intervention is required to protect the client. For instance, you might agree that you will do what is necessary while using a prearranged signal or sign, and the interpreter will interpret your explanation after the client is no longer in danger. It may be helpful to rehearse the agreed-upon strategy to determine if it will be effective and to be sure everyone understands it.

Explaining Technical Terms

Translations can proceed smoothly when the interpreter knows the subject. When the topic is not familiar, there is still little difficulty when the interpreter is transliterating word for word with a coded system (such as fingerspelling or braille). However, when the topic and terminology are unfamiliar and the interpreter must translate into another language (especially a language that does not have words for many of the terms used), interpreting may be difficult. It may help to familiarize the interpreter beforehand with the concepts that will be used or introduced during your session with the client and to describe concepts and techniques graphically, rather than rely on English and technical vocabulary (see "Communicating with People Whose Primary Language Is ASL" in this chapter and "'Pictorial Description'" in Chapter 2.)

Once the client grasps the concept or understands the technique and learns the technical term for it, the three of you may decide how to refer to that concept or technique in the future. For example, the client may prefer that the interpreter fingerspell the term, or you can all invent a sign for that term (see "'Pictorial Description'" in Chapter 2). If you use a different interpreter for another lesson, demonstrate the agreed-upon sign to the interpreter, so he or she can use it to translate to the client.

Importance of Accuracy and Impartiality

When interpreters try to explain something themselves, rather than interpret for you, you are cut out of the process. Not only must the deaf-blind person depend on the interpreter's understanding of the concept (rather than yours), it makes you less able to gauge the client's understanding so you can learn the best way to explain things to that person. When teaching some of her deaf-blind students, mobility instructor and AFB national program associate Elga Joffee had to use paraprofessional staff of schools as interpreters. She noticed that these staff sometimes used their own explanations when they thought her students did not understand what she said. She found that having to check the interpreter's accuracy made it difficult for her to concentrate on teaching the lessons.

If you do not know sign language, you may be tempted to require the interpreter to translate everything you say sentence by sentence or even word by word, so you can recognize when the interpreting is not accurate. Remember, however, that ASL is not translated literally from English, and competent interpreters often wait to hear several sentences in English before translating them into ASL. Your best clue that an interpreter is getting involved is when the interpreter answers the deaf-blind person (rather than interprets what the client said so you can respond yourself, through the interpreter). If this happens, explain to the interpreter and the deaf-blind person the necessity for an accurate, faithful rendition of everything that is communicated, so the interaction or teaching process can proceed smoothly. Of course, this clue is also useful to deaf-blind people; if they realize that the interpreter is replying to what you said without interpreting it, they may realize that they are not getting an accurate interpretation. If you do not correct this situation or if you respond directly to the interpreter, it can make clients feel left out and decrease their trust.

Establishing Trust and Rapport

Normally, when two people communicate with each other through an interpreter, they can get a clear sense of each other's personality by seeing or hearing each other while the interpreter translates. When the other person is not able to see or hear or have physical contact with you, however, it is harder for him or her to get to know you or for you to establish rapport with and gain his or her trust.

Thus it is crucial for the interpreter to convey the expression and feeling behind your messages accurately to the deaf-blind person through hand and body movements. An interpreter who is experienced in working with people who are deaf-blind should do so automatically, but some interpreters, even professionals, are not aware of how they come across when they use tactile communication. See if the interpreter's touch is conveying the feeling behind your message, such as calmness, emphasis, irritation, or empathy (see "Conveying Expression through Touch" in Chapter 2). If you speak calmly and the interpreter's hands move emphatically or if you speak emphatically and the interpreter's hands move lightly and rapidly, be aware that the client is losing an important part of the translation and that your personality and the feeling behind your messages are not being conveyed.

Another way to give the person a sense of who you are is through direct contact. Every person has his or her own level of comfort with physical contact. In working with many people who are deaf-blind, I have found that it is often considered acceptable and even desirable to hug when greeting, departing, and expressing feeling (for example, in offering support during a difficult lesson). However, some service providers and some deaf-blind people (especially those with a significant amount of remaining vision) are uncomfortable and reluctant to do so. Through the interpreter, you may ask the deaf-blind person what kind of physical contact he or she would be comfortable with—a handshake, pats on the hand or arm, or hugs—and provide as much direct contact as is appropriate and comfortable for both of you. The physical contact might take place when you guide the deaf-blind person and when you greet and take leave of him or her.

Choosing an Interpreter

The agency for which you are working with your client may provide an interpreter, or you may need to find an interpreter yourself. Most communities have private agencies that contract to provide interpreters for deaf people, and many interpreters contract individually. Agencies that serve deaf people, your deaf-blind client, the agency that referred him or her, or chapters and affiliates of the Registry of Interpreters for the Deaf (RID) in the United States and the Association of Visual Language Interpreters of Canada (AVLIC) (see Resources) may also be able to refer you to interpreter services. According to *Strategies for Serving Deaf-Blind Clients* (1984), interpreters are usually found in metropolitan areas, but there are shortages in outlying areas.

In some situations it is best to use an interpreter who specializes or is experienced in certain settings, such as classrooms, courtrooms, hospitals, or churches, or with people with minimal language skills. For example, when looking for an interpreter for O&M lessons, it would be best to find one who is experienced in that area. The next best alternative is an interpreter who has experience with deaf-blind people and is interested in O&M. If you cannot locate such an interpreter, find one who is interested in working with people who are deaf-blind.

When choosing an interpreter, consider the following issues:

1. RID and AVLIC, the certifying bodies for interpreters in the United States and Canada, certify interpreters who are skilled in interpreting ASL into spoken English, and vice versa, or in transliterating spoken English into Signed English, and vice versa.

   The interpreter should not only be skillful, but professional and impartial. Those who are certified by RID or AVLIC agree to adhere to its code of ethics. That is, they strive to convey the speaker's message (including his or her expressions) exactly in a language that the deaf person can easily understand, not to interject personal opinions or advice, and to keep all interpreting assignments strictly confidential. If the interpreter is not certified, it is important that he or she be familiar with and adhere to this code of ethics.

2. No certification has been established in the United States or Canada for interpreting for people who are deaf-blind or for verifying the interpreter's proficiency in communication methods, such as tactile signs, fingerspelling, and print on palm, that deaf-blind people use. Interpreters can attend workshops and read publications that discuss the adaptations of communication methods for deaf-blind people and acquaint interpreters with such issues as how to guide clients and the need to describe the environment to deaf-blind persons and indicate who is speaking. In Ontario, this training is offered at the Canadian National Institute for the Blind (see Resources) and George Brown College to prepare people to be "intervenors" (interpreters and guides for deaf-blind people).

   Nevertheless, many interpreters are still uncomfortable with or are not skilled in interpreting for people who are deaf-blind. DiPietro (1978, p. 6) suggested contacting the interpreter several days in advance so if "the interpreter is not familiar with the deaf-blind person's preferred mode of communication, there is time to locate an interpreter who has this particular skill." Dorothy Walt, who coordinates a program for deaf-blind people and is herself deaf-blind, observed that it may be helpful to ask the deaf-blind person to recommend interpreters with whom he or she has worked successfully because some interpreters think they are skilled in the required communication techniques of people who are deaf-blind when they are not or are not skilled in particular modes of communication.

3. If communication will be intense and prolonged, two interpreters may be necessary so they can relieve each other every 20 minutes. Tactile communication or prolonged fingerspelling can be tiring. If the communication will not be continuous, such as when the deaf-blind person will be practicing skills in addition to dialogue with the instructor, one interpreter may suffice.
4. For meetings at which there is an interpreter for other deaf people (a "platform" interpreter), deaf-blind participants who need interpreters for close-up or tactile communication can use qualified deaf people who can copy or interpret from the platform interpreter.

Using a Family Member or Friend to Interpret

It is ill advised to use the deaf-blind person's family member or friend as an interpreter for two reasons. First, such an interpreter sometimes interjects personal opinions or misconstrues the message (without your being aware of it, if you are not familiar with the language). Second, it is easier to fall into the trap of having the interpreter involved in the conversation.

I discovered that using an interpreter with a foreign-born person who does not speak English raises almost identical issues as using an interpreter for a deaf person does. Patricia Risinger, manager of TESS, a community service organization in Takoma Park, Maryland, most of whose clients are foreign born, noted (personal communication, 1991) that "messages are much more likely to be interpreted precisely through a trained and impartial third person than through a family member or friend. The relative or friend is involved in family or personal dynamics and often has a strong viewpoint, which can interfere with interpretation. It would be helpful to discuss ahead of time what the role of each person will be, so this problem can be decreased, particularly when using an untrained interpreter."

My experience with an elderly Hispanic client with a mild hearing loss and severe visual impairment may serve as an example. The client was alert and could understand speech well, but since he spoke little English, his son came to interpret during the interview. I noticed that when I talked to the client, his son often changed or added to my message. The son's intentions were good, but he had preconceived ideas of what I meant to say, and I knew enough Spanish to understand that he was not conveying my message exactly. Usually his message was something that I might have said myself. Sometimes, however, it was something I did not want conveyed, and I would say, "No, what I meant to say . . ." For instance, if I said to the client, "Through mobility training, you can learn to travel safely indoors without needing assistance," his son would say, "With this mobility training, you can learn to travel safely indoors without burdening your family." When I said, "We can go to your street and determine whether you hear well enough to cross there," his son said, "We can go to your street and show you that you can't cross because you don't hear well enough."

When the client and his son were interviewed by a professional colleague, I noticed that the professional was addressing the son rather than the client ("Let your father know that he can learn to do a lot of things for himself. Encourage him to. . . ."). The professional's messages were long, so the son listened and asked questions and occasionally turned to his father to relay what he could remember or what he thought was important about the conversation.

Because the son was not functioning as an impartial interpreter, the client had little direct communication with the professional and was getting only second-hand descriptions of what his son and the professional were saying. When I discussed this problem with my colleague later, he explained that he always tries to involve the family in interviews and wanted to speak to the son as well as to the client. He said he was "not prepared for a situation in which the son would try to wear two hats at once, which obviously couldn't work."

Some people use their young children to interpret, but here the difficulties are compounded. For example, some children are asked to interpret with physicians (one child had to tell her deaf parent that his illness was terminal) and lawyers (one Hispanic woman brought her young child to interpret between her and her divorce lawyer). However, it is unfair to involve a child in a process that can be emotional or stressful, such as O&M lessons, and better alternatives should be sought.

Knowing the principles that form the basis of effective communication is essential to more sensitive and efficient communication. Used in conjunction with the actual methods of communication explained in the next chapter, the principles outlined here can be the foundation of clear communication.

CHAPTER 2

METHODS OF COMMUNICATION

Before you consider how to communicate with the deaf-blind person with whom you will be working, it is important to remember that for the majority of adults who are deaf-blind, English is a second language. For many of these people, ASL is the only alternative for clear, full communication; a communication method that is based on English is not appropriate. Therefore, unless you are proficient in ASL, you will need an interpreter. Except for the use of interpreters and ASL, most of the methods described in this chapter are based on English.

The following section discusses the common ways of communicating with people who are deaf-blind: interpreters; sign language and sign codes; speech; spelling out words in some form; and such nonverbal communication as gestures, signals, and pictures. Although most methods can be used both to receive and express communication, some (such as print on palm) are used by deaf-blind people for receptive communication only and others (such as tape-recorded messages) are used for expressive communication only. The choice of which methods are most appropriate depends on each person's preferences, skills, and needs.

TYPES OF METHODS

Interpreters

One effective way to communicate with a deaf-blind person is to use an interpreter who is skilled in that person's method of communication (see "When Is an Interpreter Necessary?" and "Direct Communication through an Interpreter" in Chapter 1). Traditionally, a professional interpreter is used, but when working with a deaf-blind person who has minimal language skills or who uses a special communication system, you may want someone who is familiar with that person's nonverbal cues or communication system to serve as an interpreter.

ASL and Systems of English Signs

With ASL and such signed systems as Signed English and PSE, the deaf person who has a visual impairment may watch the signs (sometimes holding the signer's wrist to help track the hand) or may follow the signs tactilely with one or both hands on the signer's (see "Communication with Sign Language" in Chapter 1 and "Suggestions for Communicating" in this chapter).

Speech

Expressive Speech: Voice and Recorded Messages

Some people who are deaf-blind can speak clearly enough to be understood and some use speech as their main method of communication. After years of oral training and speech therapy, some people who were deaf before they learned to speak can enunciate well enough to be understood. People who become deaf after they have learned to talk usually retain good speech.

Kinney (1972, p. 39), a deaf-blind specialist on deaf-blindness, wrote that although "authorities state that the voices of many people who completely lose their hearing gradually tend to grow harsh, breathy, discordant," they can retain clear speech *if* they continue to speak because the same kinesthetic sense that enables a typist to know where to move the fingers without looking enables the deaf or deaf-blind person to remember how to talk. Kinney (1972, p. 40) suggested that "as a safeguard that the voice will have adequate daily exercise regardless of conversational opportunities, we should spend at least ten minutes each day reading aloud. . . . [If a friend or family member] will occasionally listen to us read and point out to us any pronunciation errors we may make, so much the better. . . . [They can also be encouraged] to bring to our attention words we habitually mispronounce in ordinary conversation."

People whose speech is not clear and who use it primarily with familiar people need to know whether the public can understand them and if not, should be prepared to use an alternative method. Some have another person record messages ahead of time on a tape recorder or a special augmentative communication device, such as the Attention-Getter, to be played back when needed (see Resources and "Preparation of Cards and Recorded Messages" in Chapter 3).

Receptive Speech: Lipreading and Hearing

Some deaf people, especially those who have residual hearing or who were taught the oral method of communication, understand others primarily by lipreading or "speech reading" (see "Who Uses Which Kind of Communication?" in Chapter 1). In addition, deaf people who understand PSE find lipreading useful to differentiate English words. Deaf-blind people who have enough remaining vision can continue to lipread. Since only 30 to 40 percent of the English language is visible on the lips (*Strategies for Serving*

Deaf-Blind Clients, 1984), a great many words cannot be positively identified when they are spoken randomly without auditory cues. When the words are spoken in context, however, skilled lipreaders can understand much of what is said. With a combination of lipreading and enough functional hearing, some people can comprehend almost everything.

The speaker should talk naturally, although those who tend not to move their lips should try to speak distinctly. I have found that people are able to read my lips better if I keep my jaw slightly open (with the teeth slightly apart), so they can see the movement of my tongue behind the teeth.

It is easier if the lipreader can view your face from below, so he or she can see your tongue moving against the roof of your mouth. Thus, if the lipreader is taller than you, tilt your head up at least enough to be facing him or her. If the lipreader is shorter than you, looking down at him or her may put your face in shadow. It is also more difficult to read your lips when you speak rapidly, use complicated and verbose sentences, or stand more than five feet from the lipreader (*Strategies for Serving Deaf-Blind Clients*, 1984).

Some people who are deaf-blind are able to hear well enough to understand speech. Often they are able to understand voices that are within certain frequencies more easily than others. However, do not assume that a person who wears a hearing aid can understand speech; many deaf people wear hearing aids to detect only environmental sounds (doorbells, telephones, and traffic, for example) or to help with lipreading. With most sensorineural hearing losses, speech is distorted. Hearing aids can amplify the sound, but the person will still hear the words as distorted. Because hearing aids amplify all sounds, background noises are louder and distracting, which makes it difficult or impossible for the wearer to hear and understand another person.

An assistive listening device sometimes alleviates this problem. With this device, a person talks into a hand-held microphone, which transmits the voice to the listener's hearing aid or to an amplifier by broadcast (FM or infrared), through an induction loop, or through a cord that connects directly into the amplifier or into the hearing aid (see Resources).

Spelling Out Words

Many people whose primary language is English prefer to communicate in English after they can no longer hear speech or lipread. Thus they use signs in English order or spell out English with some method. For example, Jeffrey Bohrman, who was born deaf and raised using English (with lipreading and speech), learned how to use signs when he became blind. However, he continues to think in English, rather than in ASL. He said that "many of the signs have many meanings, and often I think of different words from what the speaker was trying to say. That is why I sometimes understand better if I use more fingerspelling than signs" (personal communication, 1992). He also found that he understands and remembers better when communication is written for him (he reads it in braille). I have met many other people whose primary language is English and who also prefer written communication for instructions that they must remember or understand. The following are various ways people with impaired vision and hearing can spell out English.

Writing Print on Paper

Many people who are blind or visually impaired can write notes well. Some people who cannot see what they are writing use devices, such as a portable writing guide or template, and others keep their lines even by leaving a finger at the beginning of the last line. If a person's writing is not consistently clear or if the lines run into each other, you should provide feedback for improvement or encourage the person to use another method of communication.

To write notes to the public, the deaf-blind person should carry plenty of paper and a pencil or reliable pen or felt-tip pen. He or she may type or print ahead of time such things as a shopping list or directions for a taxi driver or have someone else do so. The person can also purchase or prepare cards for regular communication needs, such as getting assistance to cross streets, making purchases, or obtaining information (see "Preparation of Cards and Recorded Messages" in Chapter 3).

Reading Print on Paper or Palm

Some deaf-blind people can read print under good lighting or with a magnifier if the letters are large or thick enough and have enough contrast. Those who intend to receive communication from people using written notes should carry whatever is needed (such as paper and a marker that is thick and dark enough for them to read and for night travel, a pocket flashlight, lighted magnifier, or pen with attached light for the public to write to them).

Print can be enlarged with a closed-circuit television system (CCTV); table-top and portable models are available (see Resources). With skill and training, some people who are totally blind can use the Optacon to read print (see Resources). The Optacon is portable and enables the user to feel the shape of the letters with output at one finger while the other hand moves the scanner across the print.

A person who cannot see print can receive it tactilely if the other person uses his or her finger to write large printed capital letters on the deaf-blind person's palm. This communication method is called print on palm. To help make the letters clear, it is important to raise the finger off the palm as seldom as possible with each letter. For example, when printing an A, start at the bottom left and bring your finger up to the middle and down to the right again without taking it off the palm, then lift the finger to make the horizontal bar. (See Figure 1 for the letters used.) That way, it is less likely to be confused with the letter H, for which you raise your finger off the palm to make the two vertical strokes. Each letter takes up the whole palm and is placed over the top of the last one, with a slight pause between words (some people tap the palm with their flat hand between words or after each sentence).

Some people who become deaf-blind need a lot of practice to be able to read letters written on their palm because they cannot tell what shape the speaker's finger is tracing. It may help for them to put their hand on the speaker's drawing hand while the speaker traces the letters on their palm or for them to ask the speaker to hold their hand and use their finger to trace the letters on their palm. Sometimes people do not know the shape of print letters because they were born blind and had never learned them or because they have been using braille for so long that they forgot how the print letters are shaped; they need to learn the shapes of the print letters.

For people who lack sensitivity in the hand or have difficulty feeling the letters on the palm for some other reason, mobility instructor Mary Michaud-Cooney suggests printing the letters elsewhere on their bodies (such as on their backs or arms) or using their pointer fingers to trace letters on a table.

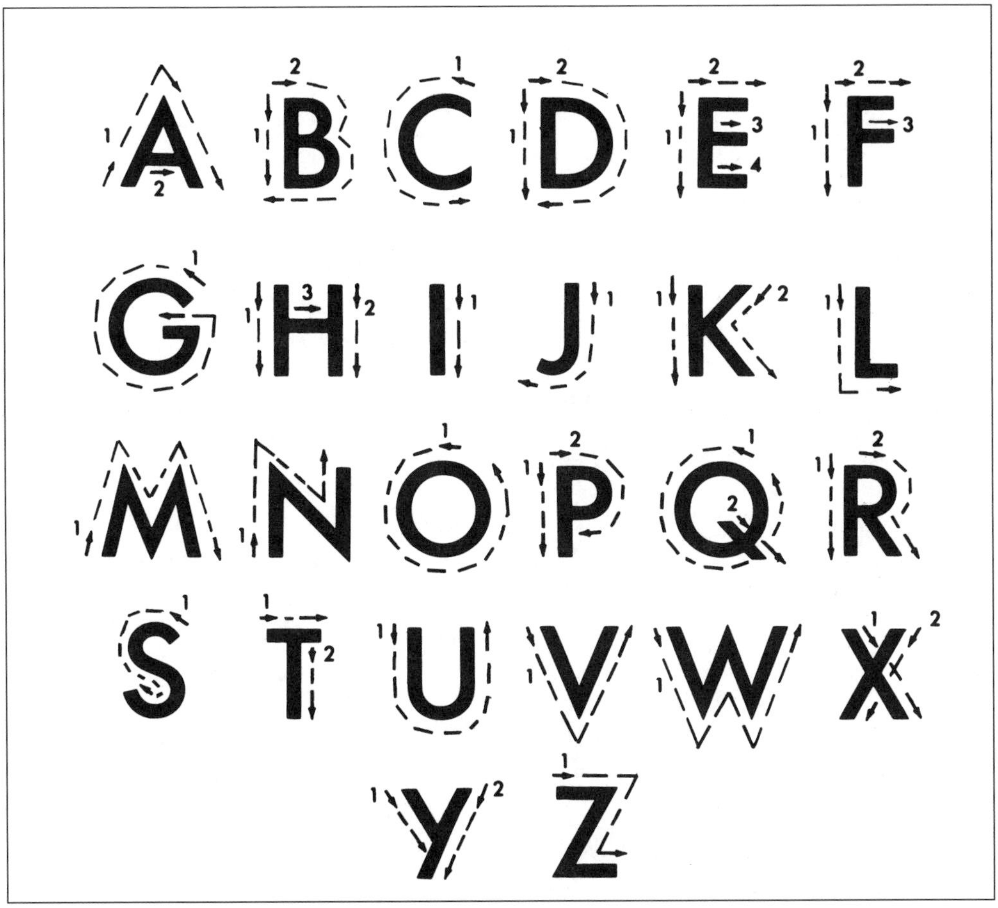

Figure 1. How to Print the Letters Used in Print on Palm. (Reprinted, by permission, from Linda Kates and Jerome D. Schein, *A Complete Guide to Communication with Deaf-Blind Persons.* ©1980 National Association of the Deaf.)

Fingerspelling

When using fingerspelling, or the American Manual Alphabet, express each letter by different shapes of the hand. (See Figure 2.) Pause between words and form each letter without moving the arm (it is difficult to read the letters if the listener has to follow the speaker's hand moving back and forth visually or tactilely). For tactile reading (feeling the shape of the hand), most people who are deaf-blind will position themselves to follow fingerspelling (see "Communication Involving Direct Touch" later in this chapter).

Two-Hand Manual Alphabets

The Two Hand Manual Alphabet, which is the predominant alphabet used by deaf-blind people in Canada, is a version of the British Manual Alphabet for the Deaf-Blind, commonly used in England. (See Figure 3.) With these alphabets, the speaker touches certain places on the deaf-blind person's outstretched hand to signify each letter. The Canadian alphabet is the same as the British one except for the letters Y and Z. Canadians start the letter Y in the same position as the British do, but they move the tip of the index finger across the receiver's palm; the Canadian letter Z is the print letter Z traced on the palm of the person receiving the message. Although few deaf-blind people in the United States know these alphabets, an increasing number of Americans have become familiar with the British Manual Alphabet because of cultural exchanges between the American Association of the Deaf-Blind and Britain's National Deaf-Blind League.

For spelling long conversations or lectures, using these alphabets is far less tiring and is faster than is using the American Manual Alphabet. They are also easier for both

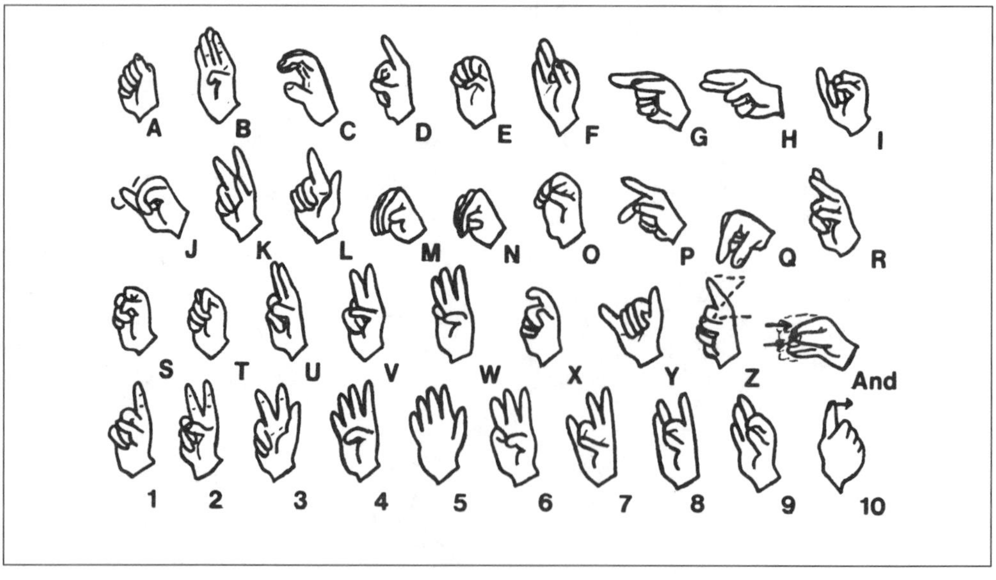

Figure 2. The American Manual Alphabet. (Reprinted, by permission, from Linda Kates and Jerome D. Schein, *A Complete Guide to Communication with Deaf-Blind Persons.* ©1980 National Association of the Deaf.)

the deaf-blind person and the speaker to learn (many can learn them in an hour). However, unlike the American Manual Alphabet and braille, which are well known in Canada and the United States because deaf people or blind people use them, these alphabets are used only with people who are deaf-blind. Thus, they are unknown except by those who communicate with deaf-blind people.

Communication Devices

There are many devices that a person can use to type messages on a keyboard and that the other person can use to read the messages in braille or print. Several devices are used primarily to communicate over the telephone or to gain access to computers, but some people who are deaf-blind also use them at work, school, or home for face-to-face written communication. For face-to-face communication, one person types on the keyboard while the other either watches the message appear on the screen or reads the braille output. A few deaf-blind travelers carry such a device for limited communication with the public, but since these devices are cumbersome, many change to print on palm or some other method after becoming proficient travelers in familiar areas. However, they bring their devices to situations where communication will be intense, such as at work or with service providers, health professionals, or friends.

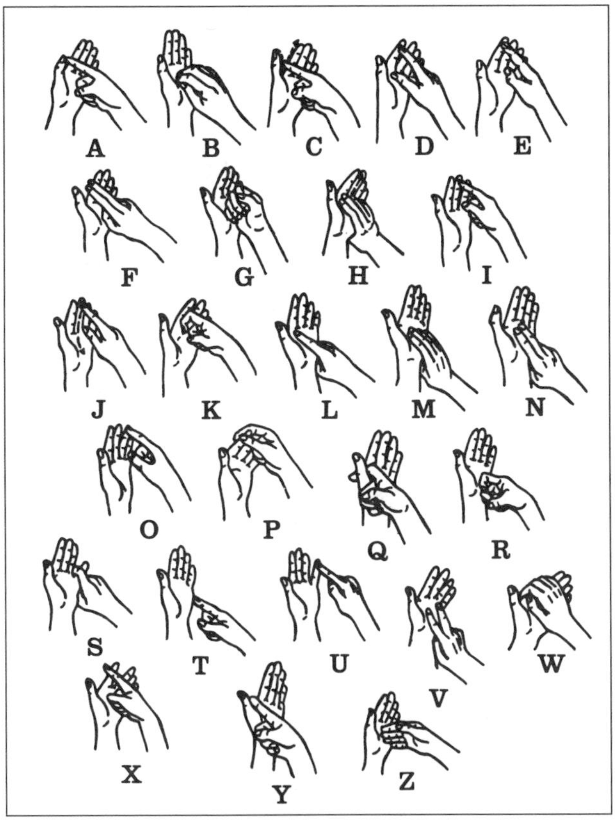

Figure 3. The British Manual Alphabet. (Reprinted, by permission, from Linda Kates and Jerome D. Schein, *A Complete Guide to Communication with Deaf-Blind Persons.* ©1980 National Association of the Deaf.)

The Alva Braille Carrier and the Teletouch are portable communication devices for deaf-blind people (see Resources). The Teletouch is a mechanical device that has one braille cell on which the deaf-blind person places his or her finger while the speaker uses a typewriter-like keyboard on the other side. Six separate keys on the keyboard can be used like a brailler to make contractions. Boyd Wolfe, who is deaf-blind, noted that when people first use the Teletouch to communicate with him, they are often confused because there is no row of numbers on the keyboard; he explains to them that they need to spell out the numbers. The Alva Braille Carrier is an electronic device that offers a braille keyboard and display on one side and a typewriter-like keyboard and print display on the other, so that the deaf-blind person and another person can type messages to each other.

Those with sufficient remaining sight can use the TDD (see Glossary), which is traditionally used to communicate over the phone to another person who has a TDD or to someone else through a relay service (see Glossary). With a normal telephone receiver placed on each TDD, one person types on the keyboard of one TDD and the message is conveyed through the telephone line to the display screen of the other TDD. For people who communicate via written notes, the TDD can also be used for face-to-face communication; one person types a message while the other reads it on the same TDD. TDD displays vary in size, color, and contrast of the letters, so people with functional vision may wish to try various models. The Superprint 100-D model can be used with an optional large-print display, which makes the letters several inches high and allows them to be displayed in various colors; several TDDs have print-out options that offer several letter sizes (see Resources). David Carrigan, who is deaf-blind, found that the screens of standard TDDs can also be seen enlarged through a CCTV, either by placing them under the CCTV camera or by connecting them to special CCTV computer equipment.

The TeleBraille II and the Infotouch are devices that connect to special TDDs and convert the letters into braille (see Resources). With these devices, the deaf person who is blind can use a TDD in the same manner that other deaf people can. Like the TDD, these devices can also be used for face-to-face communication; one person types the message while the other reads it in either print or braille.

In addition to these devices, communication in braille via computers is possible through an increasing number of technologies with refreshable braille output. With a modem, many deaf-blind braille readers use these peripheral computer attachments to communicate over the telephone with other computer users. Software is also available to use the computer to connect over the telephone with people who have a TDD rather than a computer.

Many deaf people consider it polite for the person who is answering the phone on the TDD to identify himself or herself. When finished speaking, write GA ("Go ahead") so the other person can have a turn. Do not interrupt until you see the other person write GA. When you say good-bye, write GA TO SK, meaning that you are ready to sign off. If the other person is also finished, he or she will respond with SK or SKSK. You can then type SK ("stop keying") and hang up.

Alphabet Cards or Plates

There are several boards or paper cards that have rows of print letters that can be identified by touch, either because the letters are formed with raised lines or because they are accompanied by braille letters. The speaker spells words by placing the deaf-blind person's finger on successive letters; the deaf-blind person can reply by pointing to the print letters. The Brailtalk, developed recently in Britain, is a small plastic board that folds in half and has raised-line print letters with braille beneath them. The alphabet plate is 4 inches by 6.5 inches and has raised-line print letters and numerals. According to *Strategies for Serving Deaf-Blind Adults* (1984), some people use a braille card that has braille letters underneath the printed letters.

According to Dinsmore (1959, p. 37), these devices are "a slow method of communication, but an excellent emergency device for the group who have not learned braille." Some deaf-blind people who started using the alphabet plate with the public soon abandoned it and used print on palm because they found the plate awkward to use and did not want to carry any more than necessary. These devices may be advantageous, however, when the deaf-blind person or the public prefers to avoid the physical contact that print on palm requires.

Braille Notes

Braille notes are sometimes an efficient method for communicating person to person. For one of her bright, English-literate clients, mobility instructor and AFB national program associate Elga Joffee brailled the routes, techniques, and rationale before each lesson. Jeffrey Bohrman, who is deaf-blind, found that when communication with his instructors was limited, he could understand their points better when they used braille notes and explanations. One woman with whom I worked could not receive communication effectively using any method except braille notes (see "When Communication Breaks Down" in this chapter).

During the past decade, the opportunities available to deaf-blind people who read braille have increased dramatically. Braille now provides deaf-blind people access to computers, telephones, and television (the Braille Telecaptioning System converts telecaptions into braille; see Resources). In Sweden, several technologies allow people who are deaf-blind to read the newspaper daily in braille (Lindstrom, 1990).

Communication Methods Using No Language

These methods are useful when the person who is deaf-blind wants to simplify communication, communicate with the public, or communicate while his or her hands are busy. They are also used by deaf-blind people who do not understand any standard language.

Yes-No Signals

Many people who are deaf-blind like to use quick signals for yes and no. Some tell the speaker to use one tap for yes and two taps for no (or vice versa) and three taps for "I don't know" (Dinsmore, 1959; Kinney, 1972). These signals can allow the deaf-blind person to simplify communication with both friends and the public, who often welcome such a shortcut. They can also be convenient when you are guiding a person who is deaf-blind because you can communicate by twitching your arm once for yes and twice for no (or vice versa) without interfering with the guiding. It may also be helpful for people with poor English or communication skills because they can then structure the public's response in a manner that they can control and understand. For example, they may use notes or tape recordings that ask the public to signal yes or no to specific questions prepared beforehand (with assistance, if needed).

As Rustie Rothstein, a representative of the Helen Keller National Center for Deaf-Blind Youths and Adults explained, by using a visual or tactile speech indicator, a deaf or deaf-blind person with a good speaking voice can use yes-no signals to communicate on the phone without a TDD. This technique is especially useful with services frequently used so the personnel become familiar with the technique. The deaf-blind person would ask yes-no questions ("Can you send a cab to . . . [address]?") after instructing the other person to say no, yes, and "I don't know" (or "Please repeat"). With the device, the person who is deaf-blind could feel the vibrations as the other person said one, two, or three syllables in response.

Pictures and Maps

People who are deaf-blind can communicate with the public and others by drawing or pointing to pictures or maps. Those with sufficient vision use printed material, and others can use raised-line drawings and maps (with print as well as braille for the public to understand). When a deaf-blind traveler needs to get directions, using a map can sometimes simplify things greatly.

When I teach hearing as well as deaf people who are blind, I find it effective to draw maps and shapes on their palms to explain routes, intersections, and shapes. You may use the deaf-blind person's receiving hand to sign or fingerspell what you are describing and trace the map or shape on his or her other hand. Some people also draw shapes on the deaf-blind person's back.

Deaf-blind customers who want to expedite communication or who have limited language skills can draw or point to pictures or tactile symbols of what they want to buy. These pictures or symbols can be prepared ahead of time, with the name of the item printed for the public next to the picture or tactile symbol. Pictures and symbols that are frequently used can be organized in a "communication book" that the traveler carries (see "Communicating with the Public" in Chapter 9).

Gestures and Demonstrations

Many deaf people, as well as many hearing people, use gestures to communicate a variety of things every day. We can use gestures to express our approval, concern, enjoyment, or discomfort, say hello or goodby, ask someone to leave or follow us, or indicate to a salesperson that we are ready to pay for an item. The person who cannot see the gestures of other people can feel the movement of their hands or body.

People who do not share a common language or communication system (such as deaf people and the public) can also use gestures to communicate effectively with each other. For example, deaf-blind people can use gestures to describe to a salesman what they want to buy or to indicate to a passerby their desire to cross the street. Sometimes people who have a limited grasp of language because of developmental delays or language processing difficulties can use and understand gestures.

We can also use demonstrations for effective explanations. For example, techniques can be demonstrated to the deaf-blind person, and deaf-blind travelers can demonstrate to others how to print on their palm. Again, people who cannot see a technique being demonstrated are usually able to follow the demonstration by touch.

Signals, Symbols, and Home Signs

Signals can be set up with deaf-blind people ahead of time to communicate almost anything. Some people use prearranged signals when they guide a person who is deaf-blind to indicate that the door ahead opens to the right or left or that stairs are ahead. To communicate with clients while they walk, I have used signals to indicate improvements needed in the cane technique (see "Description of Cane Movement" in this chapter and "Distance of the Instructor from the Client" in Chapter 7) and what kind of traffic is passing (see "Decisions About Crossing Without Assistance" in Chapter 8). Also, many people have their own signal or name sign so the person who is deaf-blind can identify them quickly and easily.

Symbols and object cues can be used with people whose comprehension of language is limited to enable them to express themselves and their needs. Symbols and cues can also be used to convey information to such clients (see Chapter 9, "Teaching Orientation and Mobility to People with Limited Language Skills").

Home signs are signs that are not generally recognized, but that family members or friends made up and use. Many deaf people use a few home signs that they share with others. However, the language of a few deaf and deaf-blind people is limited to such home signs, and the service provider will need to become familiar with these home signs to communicate with these clients. If possible, these deaf-blind people should learn standard signs or language systems so their communication is not limited only to those who understand their home signs (see "Communication Skills" in Chapter 9).

X Signal for Emergencies

The letter X can be traced somewhere on the deaf-blind person's body, such as the back, to indicate that there is an emergency that requires immediate cooperation. It can be done by anyone who needs to guide the deaf-blind person swiftly to safety or to give the person who is deaf-blind urgent instructions when there is no time to explain the situation. As soon as possible, the person should explain to the deaf-blind person what is happening.

This signal is not known by many people who are deaf-blind, but it should be recognized universally. Inform the deaf-blind person and those who are familiar with him or her the meaning of this signal. It would have been useful when the wing of the nursing home in which one of my clients resided had to be evacuated immediately because of an extensive gas leak. It probably would have been quickest to explain the problem to her and guide her out peacefully, but instead the nurses just grabbed her and tried to pull her out of her room. When she protested, three of them pushed her, chair and all (not a wheelchair!), into the next hall. I found her there, angry and baffled, while the staff ran to evacuate other residents. After I explained that it was an emergency and that they had no time to tell her what was happening, she understood and cooperated. She and the staff can now use this signal to indicate that there is no time for explanations and that for her safety, her cooperation is needed.

Less Common Methods of Communication

Although the following methods of conveying English are listed in other publications as being commonly used by people who are deaf-blind, few deaf-blind people with whom I am familiar use them. Nevertheless, the deaf-blind person and you may prefer to use one of them or one of the dozens of others listed in Kates and Schein (1980). As Stig Ohlson (1989), chairman of the World Blind Union's Standing Committee on Deaf-Blindness, advised other deaf-blind people at the 1989 convention of the British National Deaf-Blind League, "If the method [of communication] functions in your own environment, it does not matter if it is not used by other deaf-blind people that you never meet. . . . There is a large number of deaf-blind people who are old . . . and who do not have the strength to learn more difficult methods of communication. They have a better use for a simple method, easy to learn and easy to use. And, not least important, this method must be known to the people that surround you in your daily life."

Finger Braille

If the speaker and the person who is deaf-blind both know braille, the speaker can indicate braille letters on the deaf-blind person's body. Finger braille is used often in Japan, and it can be used to communicate rapidly. Put the first, second, and third fingers of both your hands on the corresponding fingers of the deaf-blind person. Tap or push your fingers down slightly to correspond to the braille alphabet and contractions (as if using a brailler). If you are facing the person who is deaf-blind, one of you will have to use the braille backward (as is done on a slate and stylus).

Another method is to imagine the six-dot braille cell on the deaf-blind person's palm or another part of the body. The speaker then uses a finger (or six fingers) to touch the appropriate dots for each letter. Make the imaginary braille cell large, so it is easy to distinguish where each dot is.

Alphabet Glove

To make an alphabet glove, letters are marked on any thin-fabric glove, as illustrated in Figure 4. The person who is deaf-blind memorizes the standard location of the letters, and the speaker touches each letter to form words. If the speaker has also memorized the letters, this method can be used without the glove and, with practice, it can be fast.

Raised-line Drawings and Letters

Some people who cannot see print and do not know braille or whose sensitivity in the fingers is reduced so they cannot read braille may be able to use letters or drawings made with raised lines. You can draw raised lines by placing plastic sheets or thick paper on a soft surface, such as heavy cardboard or a braille book, and write or draw backwards. When you turn the paper over, the lines will be raised. Make the lines deep enough and the letters and shapes large enough to be discerned. Commercial materials for making raised lines are also available, as well as machines that produce raised-line copies of inkprint letters and drawings (see Resources). If the plastic sheets can hold the raised lines permanently, the deaf-blind person can keep telephone numbers or other information on them.

Plastic Letters

The person who is newly blind and deaf may understand words formed with the plastic letters sold at toy stores. Stig Ohlson (1989) said, "At the time I lost my sight and my hearing, I started to use large plastic letters to receive information. It was slow, but it was a means to get in touch with people around me again. It was an exact method, and it was easy for everyone to use. I soon left this method because it was too slow, and because it demanded that you were comparatively settled. But it had its advantages as long as I needed it."

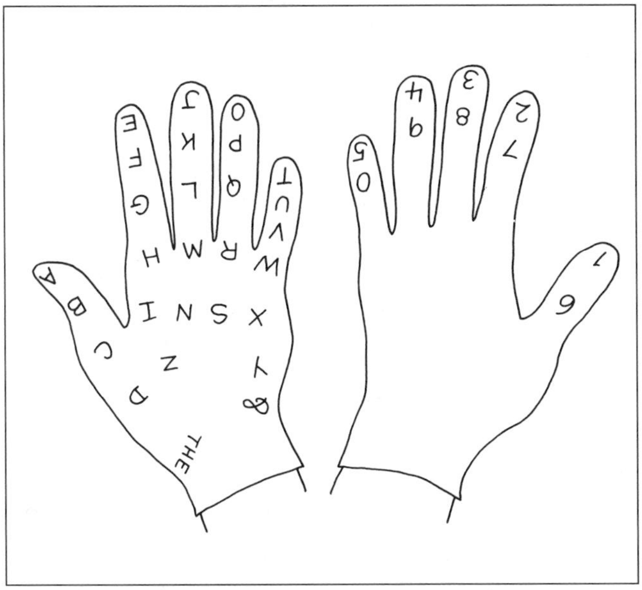

Figure 4. The Alphabet Glove. (Reprinted, by permission, from Linda Kates and Jerome D. Schein, *A Complete Guide to Communication with Deaf-Blind Persons.* ©1980 National Association of the Deaf.)

Morse Code

If both people know the Morse code, it can be tapped onto the deaf-blind person's hand or other part of the body. This method, as well as printing large block letters on other parts of the body, may be useful for the diabetic deaf-blind person who lacks enough sensitivity in the hands to use other methods of communication. It can also be used to communicate over the telephone if the deaf-blind person can detect the sounds as the other person voices or taps the signals.

Tadoma

A deaf-blind person using the Tadoma method places his or her thumb lightly on the lips of the speaker to feel breath sounds (for sounds such as s, f, ch, and sh) and lip movement (to tell vowels from consonants and diphthongs). The index finger is placed along the side of the nose to detect nasal sounds (m, n, and ng), and the other fingers are placed on the cheek and throat to detect voiced consonants that vibrate (such as b, d, and z).

Although many people object to having a stranger put a hand on their lips, this method can be effective. It allows the person who is deaf-blind to understand much of what is said. Those who are skilled with Tadoma use it primarily with family members and friends.

Although the literature often cites Tadoma as a method of communication for deaf-blind people, only a handful of people who are deaf-blind know how to use it. According to Dinsmore (1959), it takes years of training to learn this method, and the deaf-blind people who use it learned it during early childhood. One of those people, Robert J. Smithdas, said that he knows of only six living deaf-blind people who use Tadoma. He thinks that although the method is not obsolete, teachers today do not take the time that is required to teach it. Jeanne Prickett, a consultant on deaf-blindness, added that one reason that Tadoma is not taught may be because the instructional methods have not been well documented or disseminated. The only person alive of whom Smithdas is aware who has taught it is the retired speech teacher who taught him at the Perkins School for the Blind.

According to Smithdas, Tadoma was named after the first children to learn the Vibration Method—"Tad" Chapman, who is now in his 80s, and a girl named Oma, who died in her 30s. It is still sometimes suggested that deaf-blind children place a hand on the speaker's face in the Tadoma position to become aware that others are using their voice to communicate (California State Department of Health, 1974), but Smithdas knows of no one who is actually teaching people to understand speech by using the Tadoma method.

SUGGESTIONS FOR COMMUNICATING

This section offers suggestions for using various methods of communication with deaf-blind persons. The most important suggestion, however, would be to find out from the person what makes the interaction easiest for him or her. Deaf-blind people should be encouraged to inform others of their communication needs.

Communication Involving Direct Touch

There are many methods by which people can receive communication tactilely, including print on palm, fingerspelling, sign language, the British Manual Alphabet, finger braille, and the alphabet glove. To initiate communication tactilely with deaf-blind people, contact them on the hand, arm, or shoulder to avoid startling them. If you need to touch them somewhere else (for example, to point to something on their clothes or face) or to touch something they are holding, let them know what you are doing. I usually put my hand under theirs and then bring my hand toward them with their hand on mine, so they realize that I am about to touch them.

Sometimes it can be awkward to communicate tactilely without scratching the deaf-blind person. Keep your fingernails short and smooth and avoid large or sharp rings. You can soften rough, dry hands with lotion, but do not leave your hands greasy. In warm environments, carry a small container of powder to shake over your hands whenever the communication gets sticky. In winter, a "mobility muff" can make conversations in freezing weather comfortable (see Appendix A for instructions).

Techniques

To initiate tactile sign language or tactile fingerspelling, put your hand or hands under those of the person who is deaf-blind. Some people, especially those who are learning sign language or tactile communication, will need to put both their hands on yours as you sign, but experienced people generally use only one hand, placed on your dominant signing hand. When it is important that you describe something using both your hands, put your hands under both of theirs.

Just sign as you normally would. If people choose to follow your signs with only one hand, they can feel your hand move and touch your other hand for most signs. However, remember that since much of ASL requires facial expressions and body language, if the person cannot see your face or body, this information must be conveyed through the hands. For example, you can use the sign for "not," rather than shake your head, and the sign for "question", rather than a quizzical expression.

To maximize the communication between you and the deaf-blind person, make sure that the two of you are comfortable. As mobility instructor William VanBuskirk pointed out, it is difficult for some people to get used to having a deaf-blind person's hand over theirs as they fingerspell or sign. Many people who are deaf-blind have different styles—some are heavy on the signer's hand, and others are light. Let the deaf-blind person know if the communication is uncomfortable or awkward for you; perhaps it would be better if he or she would use a lighter touch or assume a different position. Likewise, some deaf-blind people who use fingerspelling prefer to have their hand over the back of the other person's hand, others prefer that the other person faces them and fingerspells into their cupped hand, and still others hold the signer's wrist (to help follow the signs visually or to feel the movement of tendons and muscles in the hand). For long fingerspelling sessions, it is less fatiguing if both of you can rest your elbows on a table or on the arm of a chair or even on your knees.

Some people understand fingerspelling that is lightly pressed into their palms. When fingerspelling into the cupped palm of others, however, place important fingers prominently into their hand. For example, the letters G, H, M, and N are formed with protruding fingers; to form those letters, I put the protruding fingers between the person's thumb and first finger. I sometimes lightly squeeze the two or three fingers that distinguish the letter N from M onto the person's thumb.

When signing, bring your hand (with the deaf-blind person's hand on top) to the proper place on your body; do not move your body to accommodate the sign. Some signs (for example, for "father," "mother," and "fine" and for "fun" and "cute") are similar except for the placement on the speaker's body. If a person signs "fun" (signed on the nose) by bringing the face down to the hand, the person who is deaf-blind may think the sign is being made lower on the face, confusing it with the sign for "cute" (signed on the chin).

Conveying Expression Through Touch

> There is no need to speak; I understand
> each quick impulsive movement of your hand.
> By some strange magic of the heart I guess
> the meaning of each gesture, each caress.
>
> Your fingers can be gentle, firm, or kind;
> or fierce when anger surges through your mind.
> Or they can trace, with such exquisite grace,
> the tenderness love mirrors in your face.
>
> Oh, when I reach to take you by the hand,
> it is because I need to understand
> that I am not alone in this broad land.
> —"Touch" in Smithdas, *Shared Beauty* (1982), p. 46.

Normally, we convey our feelings with our facial expression and tone of voice. With tactile communication, feelings are conveyed through the hands and body. The poem "Touch," whose author is deaf-blind, expresses this fact beautifully. Helen Keller's description of her encounter with George Bernard Shaw, who was her hero, also shows how strongly those impressions can come through: "I held out my hand. He took it indifferently. I could scarcely believe my sensations. Here was a hand bristling with egotism as a Scotch thistle with thorns. It was not the sort of hand that one would associate with the compassionate interpreter of Joan of Arc" (quoted in Lash, 1980, p. 642).

Whether signing, fingerspelling, or printing on palm, your hands can express different moods. Slow, smooth movements may convey calm or confidence; fast, emphatic movements may convey urgency or authority; light, mischievous movements may convey playfulness; and tentative movements may convey shyness or uncertainty. I sometimes express impatience by drumming my fingers on top of the deaf-blind person's hands or by placing my fist on my waist while the person's hand is on mine. I may show empathy by using slow, smooth signs or stroking or patting the person's hand. Char Laba, who coordinates services for deaf-blind people, noted that guesswork can be eliminated if you describe facial expressions or moods directly ("I am laughing" or "I feel sad").

Your body can also convey expression as you guide the deaf-blind person or stand or sit close enough to be in contact. After congratulating a client who has done an outstanding job on a lesson, I sometimes swagger proudly as we walk back to the car. When a person teases me while his or her hand is on mine, I may mockingly shake my fist or, bringing my hand to my chin so the person can feel where my head is, I put my face almost against the person's. If we are walking when someone teases me, I may walk stiffly, bristling "in a huff" (sometimes having to assure the person I am also just teasing). I once showed my exasperation with one man by putting his hand on my shoulder as I slowly sank to the floor (he laughed and apologized). To clarify the situation and keep the deaf-blind person from guessing, you may also give the sign for "ha-ha-ha" or "teasing you!" with your statement.

No doubt, you will come up with your own ways of expressing yourself and conveying your own unique personality. Since deaf-blind people cannot see your response as they communicate, it helps if you respond during the conversation with appropriate signs, such as "yes" or "I see" or "ha-ha-ha."

When the Person Sees Sign Language

When communicating with people who use vision, wear solid-color clothing that contrasts with your skin. Dorothy Walt, who is deaf-blind, suggests that black, navy blue, and dark blue clothes are best for light-skinned people (avoid reds and oranges), and white and yellow are best for dark-skinned people (the light colors should not be so bright as to cause glare). You can bring a shirt or jacket or tie-on vest of the appropriate color to wear over your clothes, if necessary. Avoid distracting jewelry. Make sure the lighting is good for the person who is deaf and visually impaired. The light should be in front of your body, and there should be no glare from windows or lights behind you.

A common misconception among people who live or work with people with restricted visual fields is that "tunnel vision" is shaped like a tunnel when it is actually shaped like a cone or funnel. That is, the farther the person is from another person or object, the more of that person or object is in view. Ask the person what is the best distance for you to stand, and find out the size of the person's visual field at the distance from which you are signing; then you can either make your signs in an area small enough to fit within that visual field or move farther away where he or she can see more of you. In any case, keep the signs close to your face (but not in front of your mouth), so the person can see your facial expression and read your lips while watching your signs.

Some people who have retinitis pigmentosa, diabetic retinopathy, and several other eye diseases require 10 to 30 minutes to adjust to changes in light. If they are going into bright light from a dark area, or vice versa, allow them time to adjust and ask them to let you know when they can see your signs again. In the meantime, you may use sign language tactilely (see "Adjusting to a New Method of Communication" in this chapter).

When the Person Sees Print

Find out what size print the person needs and how thick the letters must be and use an appropriate-size dark pen or marker on white- or light-colored paper. If notes must be read where lighting is not adequate, be prepared with appropriate portable lighting (such as a flashlight during a night lesson). Deaf-blind people should have an appropriate magnifier ready if needed. If they intend to communicate with the public by having other people write notes, they should carry not only paper, but whatever markers the public should use to write, as well as any lights and magnifiers that will be needed to read the notes.

When the Person Lipreads or Understands Speech

When the person lipreads, ask at what distance you should stand for him or her to read your lips. The lighting should be on your face, not from behind where it leaves your face in shadow.

When the person understands speech auditorily, speak clearly and naturally and ask where you should stand and at what volume you should speak. For many people who use hearing aids, loud voices can be painful, since the hearing aid already amplifies the sound. Some people can understand voices in certain frequencies better than in others, so ask the person if it is better if you speak with a lower or higher tone of voice. Try to talk in areas with little or no background noise; when you need to talk in noisy areas, try an assistive listening device (see "Receptive Speech: Lipreading and Hearing" in this chapter).

Notes and Communication Devices

When communicating with such methods as written or brailled notes or communication devices, it is hard to be expressive. Dinsmore (1959, p. 7) compared mechanical communication devices to other methods: "Psychologically, it has been found that the touch of hand upon hand establishes a rapport similar to that developed through auditory or visual stimuli. For the deaf-blind, the hand takes the place of a smile or tone of voice. If however, a device can overcome the reluctance of the general public to attempt conversation with deaf-blind people, it will have served an invaluable purpose."

Anyone communicating by phone with a TDD experiences the same difficulty in being warm and personal. People try to overcome this problem by inserting expression during a conversation with such phrases as "smile," "hahaha," "ugh!" "grin," "wink," "ahem!" "hug," "hmmm," "sigh!" and "grrr!" These expressions may help when using mechanical communication methods with deaf-blind people as well. For example, one may type into the Teletouch, "It is good to see you again [pause] smile [pause] are you ready for another lesson [pause] I thought we'd try to walk to China today haha." When communicating through notes or mechanical devices, try to make up for the lack of a personal touch by letting your personality come through in other ways.

COMMUNICATION CODES

TDD Abbreviations:

ANS:	Answer
CUD:	Could
GA:	Go ahead (your turn)
HD:	Hold
LTR:	Letter
MSG:	Message
MIN:	Minute
NITE:	Night
PLS:	Please
Q (or QQ):	? (leave space before the Q)
R:	Are
REC:	Received
SK:	Good-bye (stop keying)
U:	You
UR:	Your
WUD:	Would

There are some abbreviations that people customarily use on the TDD, such as "pls" (please) and "U" (you) (see "Communication Codes" for some of these abbreviations, as well as abbreviations for courtesies and conventions when using the TDD). These abbreviations may be confusing for those who use both braille and TDD; I sometimes mistakenly use a TDD abbreviation for a braille contraction, and vice versa.

WHEN COMMUNICATION BREAKS DOWN

When there is poor communication between you and the deaf-blind person, it may be because the communication method is not being used well enough or the deaf-blind person needs better lighting or quieter circumstances. For example, perhaps you are talking too loudly or too softly or not clearly enough to a person who is hard-of-hearing. Perhaps the letters that you are printing on the deaf-blind person's palm are not sufficiently large or clear. For the person who sees signs, perhaps you are making the signs too close or in too large an area for his or her reduced visual field or too far away to be seen clearly. In these cases, you should find out from the deaf-blind person or others who know the person how best to communicate with him or her. Flexibility and sensitivity are important. Figures 5A and B show how an instructor can optimize the communication environment for the client. Here the instructor wears clothing of solid color that contrasts with her hands, begins in a well-lit area where one of the hall lights illuminates the front of her, and shifts communication methods under poorer lighting conditions.

Other factors can contribute to a breakdown in communication. Sometimes the service provider uses a communication method that is based on English and does not realize that the person understands only ASL. If this is the case, an ASL interpreter is needed.

Occasionally, the worker uses the wrong method of communication. Once when I was asked to orient a deaf-blind college student to her new campus, I was told that she could speak well, but that her receptive communication skills were poor. I observed that when the college personnel communicated with her, she recognized only about 10 signs and was able to read fingerspelling at the rate of only about one word a minute. When I started orienting her, she verbally asked yes-no questions about the routes, but I was frustrated because I was unable to use signs or fingerspelling to explain anything to her. After a while, however, I realized that she was able to understand me well if I spoke distinctly within a few inches of her left ear. Needless to say, once I'd found her preferred method of communication, the orientation went smoothly.

However, if you are skillfully using a method that the deaf-blind person can normally understand, the problem may be that he or she is losing the vision or hearing needed to use that method of communication and must use another method (such as tactile communication or an assistive listening device). If the deaf-blind person becomes defensive and blames you or the interpreter for the communication problem, be patient, do not take it personally, and ensure the person that you will not abandon him or her because of the effort and time required to communicate. As Primrose-McGowan (1980, p. 1) wrote about this stage, "Patience and ingenuity are needed

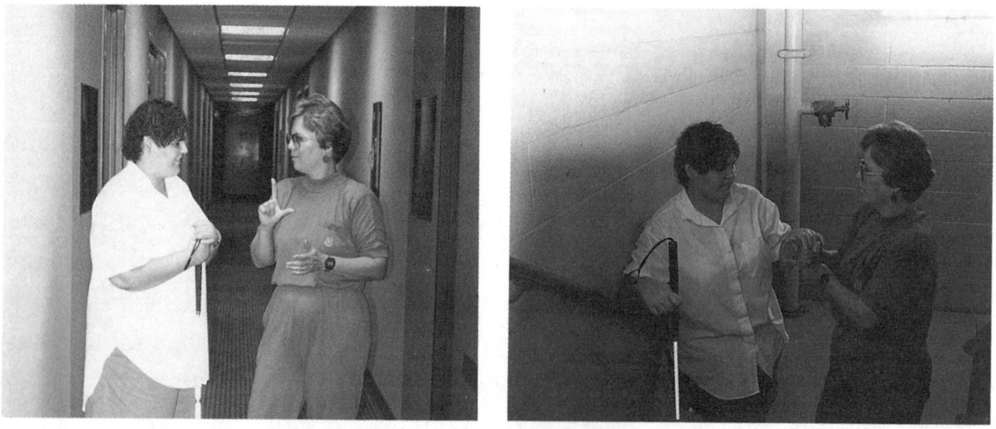

Figures 5A and B. This deaf visually impaired woman can see the instructor's signs in well-lit areas. In dark areas, however, the woman follows the instructor's signs by placing her hand on that of the instructor.

since the channels of effective communication are frequently not immediately open, and at times, the instructor's expectations of the trainee's performance may be too great."

Adjusting to a New Method of Communication

For most deaf people who relied on sign language before they lost their vision, the transition to tactile sign language is comparatively easy, although as Caryn Spall, who is deaf-blind, pointed out, the person must first adopt a positive attitude about making the change. Stig Ohlson (1989), chairman of the World Blind Union's Standing Committee on Deaf-Blindness, wrote, "In our experience, active deaf-blind people adjust more or less automatically. If they can, they use their sight to read the signs, and if they cannot, they resort to touch." For deaf people who relied on lipreading, the transition is more difficult because they must learn sign language or a method to continue to receive English (such as braille, tactile fingerspelling, or print on palm) or both.

In my experience, people who relied on hearing have the most difficulty making the transition when they become deaf-blind, although some eventually adjust well. They (and those around them) learn new methods of communication and become active and involved again with their family members, friends, community, and work.

However, some people who relied on hearing, including four with whom I worked, were not able to do so. Three of these people had been blind, and one was losing vision and hearing at the same time. Two women were proficient braille users before they lost their hearing and were able to make some adjustments. One of them was exposed to print on palm and such devices as the Teletouch and TeleBraille early enough to use them effectively, but the staff at her nursing home was unable or unwilling to use those methods. She withdrew into her own world, hallucinating often (see "Hallucinations" in Chapter 5).

The other woman had lacked any good receptive communication for so long that she would talk incessantly and hallucinated often. In one respect, she was typical of people who prefer to dominate the conversation because they have difficulty understanding others, but she carried it to the point where she was reluctant to allow others to communicate with her at all. When she was first learning to use the Teletouch, she would read a few words, then pull her hand off and start talking. In response, I would hand her a note that I had brailled saying, "I'm not done talking yet—please put your finger back on the Teletouch." This approach seemed to work, so I left the note with the staff at her nursing home. She did not improve much, however, and during her lessons I had to braille most of what I wanted to say on paper, rather than use the Teletouch. That was the only way she would finish reading a whole sentence or paragraph before pulling her hand off and responding.

The other two people did not learn new methods of communication. They preferred to communicate with their residual hearing, although it was inadequate. Even when people talked directly into their ear as clearly as possible, they still misunderstood most of what was being said. They were frustrated with or were unable or unwilling to learn print on palm, sign language, or braille. One woman who lived alone became depressed and more and more withdrawn, and she refused services several times. I do not know if she was ever able to overcome this depression and to learn a more effective method of communication. Although the other person was able to learn a few signs, his communication is still limited. He often withdraws into himself and has an active imaginary life that he seems to believe is real.

People who lose their vision or hearing slowly often are frustrated about the process of adjustment. It seems that just as they learn to function well, their vision or hearing deteriorates further, and they have to adjust once again and learn new skills for communication, daily living tasks, and mobility.

The gradual modifications that need to be made by people who rely on sign language and who have Usher's syndrome are typical examples. At first these people require sufficient light to communicate because they cannot see well in dim areas. As their visual field decreases, good lighting is not enough; they also need the other person to reduce the area of his or her signs or to be far enough away so they can see the signs. When their field of vision is severely restricted, many prefer to hold the wrist of the signer, so they know where to look for his or her hand and visually track it as it makes the signs. When they can no longer see effectively, they place their hand on the hand of the speaker and follow the signs tactilely.

A similar process of adjustment can occur when the hearing loss is slow. A woman who was interviewed by Yoken (1979, p. 65) described her experiences as follows: "At first, the hearing loss sneaks up on you and you don't believe it's really happening. Singing off key and not really sure why. . . . It became frustrating. It got increasingly difficult to hear in class. But then I'd get a better hearing aid and I'd be back in business again." Each time, the hearing aid was stronger than the one before, and she had to teach herself to identify the sounds that she had forgotten while those sounds had been inaudible. With these adjustments, she could communicate well in one-to-one situations, but not in groups or in places where there was background noise.

Working with People Who Are Learning a New Method of Communication

When you want to provide services to people who are in transition between methods of communication, how do you communicate with them? I usually use the method with which they are most comfortable and use the new method only when necessary until they become proficient in it because I believe that during our sessions, the person's concentration should be on what we are doing, rather than on the method of communication. As soon as the person is comfortable with the new method, I use it predominantly. Frequently, when we are working together, the person's proficiency in the new method is also improving, and it usually does not take long for him or her to be able to use it well.

For example, when I teach O&M, I begin each lesson where it is comfortable to communicate, so we can discuss as much as possible before the lesson begins. For night lessons with people who cannot communicate well in dark areas, we first have our discussion indoors or (if they can see my signs from nearby) in the car with the light on. During the lesson, if possible and *if* it will not jeopardize the lesson, I guide the client to a place where communication will be more comfortable (for example, a well-lit place for the client who uses vision or a quiet place for the client who uses hearing). If it is important not to disturb the lesson (such as when the client is lost and needs to practice reorienting independently) so that we must communicate in a place where the client needs to use tactile communication, I allow enough time, try to put the client at ease, and communicate slowly.

On rare occasions, if the communication is severely restricted and the client is having difficulty learning a new method of communication (as was the case with several hearing people who could no longer understand speech), I wait to begin the training until the client is more comfortable with the new method because it would be frustrating to the client, communication would be too limited, and progress would be slow. Usually, however, if the client is motivated to learn, I proceed with training. The lack of control over one's life is a major loss, and the sooner the client can learn the skills to live independently and communicate comfortably, the better. The ability to accomplish daily tasks independently can greatly increase confidence and improve the outlook of a person who is undergoing a traumatic change. Also, the desire to communicate with the practitioner can itself be an incentive to learn the new communication method faster.

When working with people whose communication is slow, allow for the extra time needed to communicate everything that would normally have been conveyed and expect that progress will be slower. As is true of any client, before you begin activities for which they need to communicate with the public, be sure that they are relatively comfortable with a method that they can use with other people.

"PICTORIAL DESCRIPTION"

For many years, when I worked only occasionally with deaf-blind people, I tried to translate the English words I normally needed to teach O&M into signs. I found, however, that I often had to fingerspell because many words and common mobility terms (such as *curb, sidewalk, cane,* and *square off*) have no equivalent in sign language. My clients usually could understand what I was explaining, but it was awkward. One deaf-blind client asked me to stop describing so much and let her explore.

Mobility instructors have told me that they, too, had trouble using signs and sign language to explain things. One instructor said she found it difficult to convey such complex techniques as the three-point touch technique to her deaf-blind client. Some suggested that we make up and agree on some signs for mobility terms that we could use when teaching deaf people and distribute the list to mobility instructors. According to Battison (1980), many teachers and other service providers who work with deaf children and adults have the same problem and either fingerspell the words or make up signs. However, she stated that these signs should be invented only as a last resort, after first studying how deaf people use signs in a conversational context and the details of how natural signs are formed.

The reason that we were frustrated is that we were trying to translate English word for word into signs, so we could describe things to deaf-blind people the same way that we do with hearing-blind people—through words. After I took several sign language classes, I had learned some signs and phrases for everyday conversation, but I still did not know how to apply them to teaching O&M. I persisted in translating more or less literally from English (PSE) because I did not know any better.

However, after watching numerous descriptions by people who are proficient in ASL, I realized that there is another way to give explanations—which I call "pictorial description"—that is more effective than English for many people. With pictorial description you describe objects, movements, and positions of the body and cane as ASL users do, using your hands to represent objects and people.

Although pictorial description is a component of ASL, it can be used regardless of whether you and the deaf-blind person use sign language or English, whether either of you know any signs, or whether the deaf-blind person receives communication visually or tactilely. I have found that sometimes even hearing-blind people and deaf-blind people who do not know how to sign can understand a certain concept or technique better when I illustrate it with my hands than when I explain it in English. Pictorial description was indispensable when I taught a hearing man from Russia who had lost his vision and spoke little English.

For example, to describe a cane technique to a person who does not sign, I explain that I will illustrate the technique by representing the cane with my finger. With his or her hands on mine, the client then feels how my finger is moving along my other hand, illustrating how the cane tip is to be moved along the ground.

In ASL, the positions or movements of objects and people can be described by classifiers, which are signs that represent an object or person. Often, the classifier for an object is not the same as its standard sign. For example, the sign for car (or *drive*) is to move the arms as if turning the steering wheel (see Figure 6). You would use that sign to say, "Let's get into the car" or "This car needs to be fixed." The classifier that can represent a vehicle, such as a car, truck, or bicycle, is shown in Figure 7. You can represent the movement or position of vehicles with one or both of your hands in the shape of this classifier.

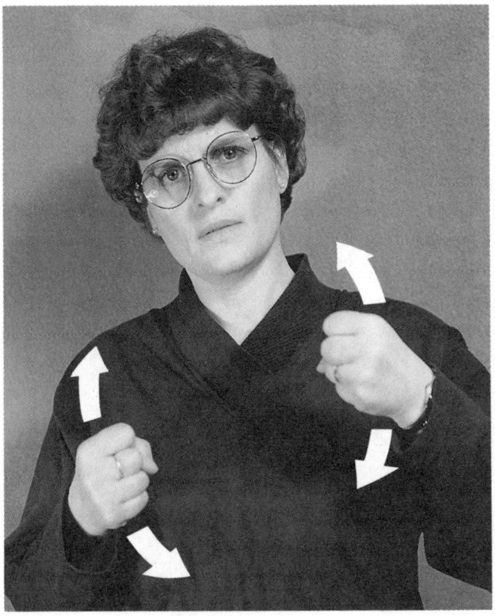

Figure 6. The sign for "car."

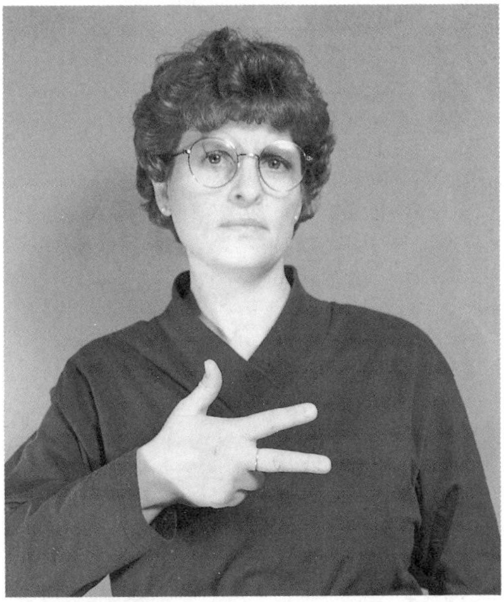

Figure 7. The classifier for a vehicle, such as a car, truck or bicycle.

Many people will learn best from a combination of actual demonstrations, pictorial description, and explanations in English or sign language (or both). For instance, I used all these methods to teach the three-point touch cane technique to one deaf-blind client. He followed all my signs and explanations tactilely (with one or both of his hands over mine). First, I explained in sign language the purpose of the technique and fingerspelled the term.

I decided to demonstrate the technique next. Using sign language, I asked him to stand next to the curb with his cane against it and explained that I would place my hand over his and move the cane while he walked along the curb, as shown in Figure 8. After we did this, he did not understand the technique, because, as he later explained, he did not understand where the tip of the cane was when I moved his hand.

I then illustrated the technique using pictorial description. My finger represented the cane, showing how it moves in relation to the curb, which I explained would be represented by my other hand (held flat). With my finger slanted at the angle that the cane would be, the tip of the finger "cane" touched the top of the "curb" (my other hand), pivoted to the side to where the street would be (in the air), slid back so the "cane" could hit the side of my hand (the "curb"), and went back up to the top to repeat the pattern, as shown in Figures 9 A-C. The client then understood what to do and practiced it. He had difficulty getting the rhythm, so I repeated the pictorial description, with my finger emphasizing the unusual rhythm required for this technique. He then tried it again while I helped him move the cane in rhythm. After practicing it once more on his own, he could do it well.

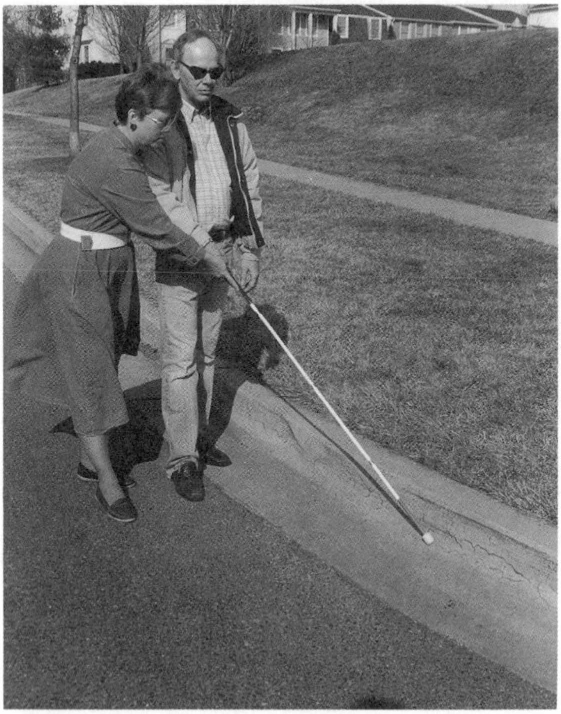

Figure 8. To teach the three-point touch technique, the instructor can demonstrate what is done by placing his or her hand over that of the client.

After the client grasps the concept, the two of you can agree on a sign that you can use in the future to refer to that concept if you do not want to spell it out. For example, a useful sign for three-point touch technique may be to move your finger in this technique against your other hand as was just described.

Some suggestions for using pictorial description are presented in the pages that follow, and you can come up with others to suit your needs. If you plan to take a sign language course, take a class in ASL, which usually teaches this skill, rather than a class in Signed English. In one popular exercise, for example, two students sit facing each other at a table. A short barrier allows each to see the other's face but not what is on the table. Both students have the same set of Tinkertoys, and one student makes an arrangement with his or her set. Without using words or even signs, that student must depict how the pieces are arranged by demonstrating and describing them using only his or her hands, so the partner can duplicate the arrangement.

Exercises such as this can help you learn to make pictures, not words, to describe the environment and mobility terms. When possible, watch a proficient

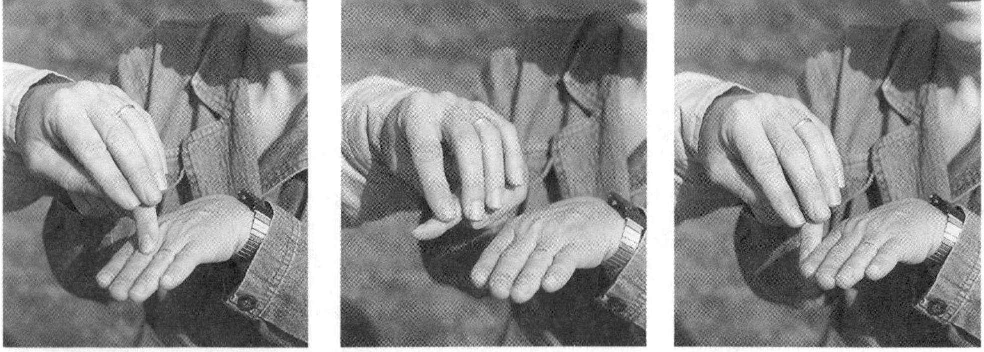

Figures 9A, B, and C. To illustrate the three-point touch technique further for the client, the instructor can use pictorial description.

ASL user describe things, then try it yourself with feedback. Though you may use any hand shape to get your point across, if you are trying to use ASL, you will need to learn the proper classifiers (see Humphries, Padden, & O'Rourke, 1980, for commonly used ASL signs and classifiers).

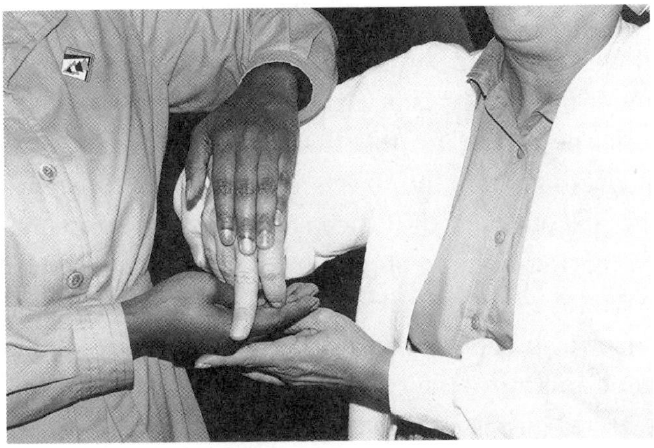

Figure 10. Using the client's hand as the "passive" hand. The movement and position of an individual at the edge of a stairway is made clear by using the palm of the deaf-blind person to represent the landing.

For many of the descriptions that follow, there is an "active" hand and a "passive" hand. When you use sign language, the active hand makes the sign or represents the object or person and sometimes acts upon the passive hand. For example, when you describe the three-point touch cane technique, the hand with the finger representing the cane is the active hand, and the hand representing the curb is the passive hand.

For some of these descriptions, people using tactile communication may need to place both hands on your hands. When they cannot tell what your active hand is doing to your passive hand (such as sliding along it for the constant-contact cane technique or "walking" along it to demonstrate the proper position for starting to descend stairs), you may have them hold out their own hand to be the passive hand. They would then place their other hand on your active hand while you move it or slide it against their passive hand. (See Figure 10.)

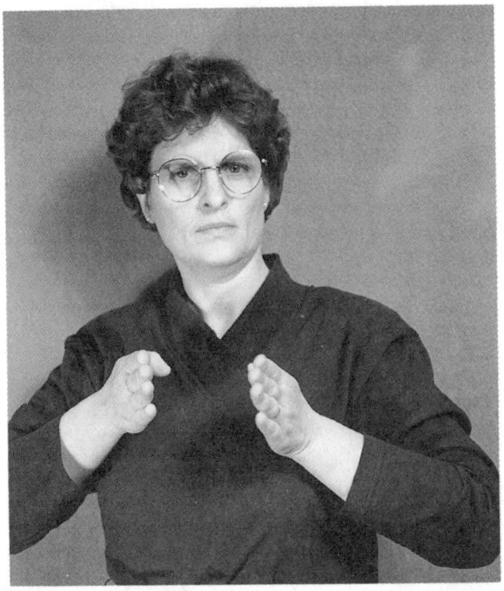

Figure 11. Describing the shape of a room.

Description of the Environment

To describe a room, explain what you are going to do, then use both hands to demonstrate the shape of the room as if it were a box in the air in front of you. (See Figure 11.) Now that you have the room represented, you can fill in the details right in the "room" that you made in the air. Doors and windows of the real room are "drawn" in the "walls" of the imaginary room. The sign for "chair" or "sit" is to bend two fingers over two fingers of the passive hand (like the legs of a person sitting). Chairs and benches and couches in the real room can be designated with just the two bent fingers placed in the imaginary room. If you are standing in the room while describing it, rather than show their location in the imaginary room, you may prefer to point to the objects themselves (windows or tables), spell or sign what they are, and outline their shape in the air toward where the real items are.

Outside, point to objects and "position" them in the air the same way. Show the width of a pole by making an appropriate circle (use your thumb and finger in a C shape if the pole is narrow and both hands, each in the form of a C, if the pole is wide and move the circle up or down to signify "pole"). A rounded curb may be depicted by a hand with the fingers bent 90 degrees and moving around in the shape of the curb (see Figure 12). Illustrate the position of walls with your flat hand moving in the direction of the wall. Two flat hands moving perpendicular to each other can meet to show where the corner is, or one hand can move one way then turn, to represent the corner.

To show two sidewalks or streets in relation to each other, represent each one with an index finger. Place your fingers horizontal to the ground, since they are representing horizontal streets. The fingers can approach and cross each other to represent an intersection. A T intersection can be shown by the tip of one finger coming perpendicular to the middle of the other finger, forming a T. Fingers moving parallel to each other can represent parallel streets or sidewalks or can move toward each other at an odd angle to represent an unusual intersection.

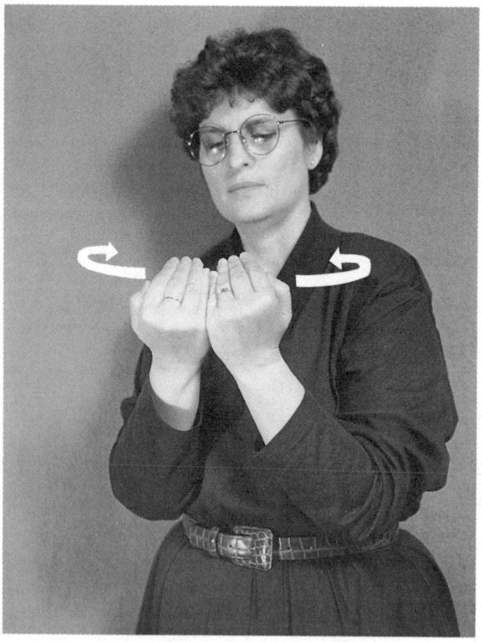

Figure 12. Describing a rounded curb.

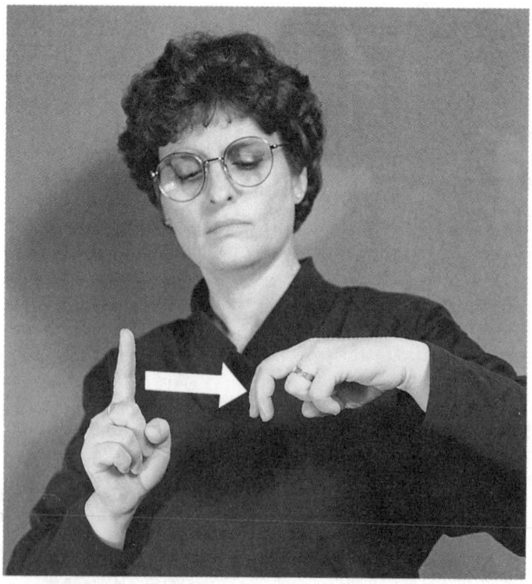

Figure 13. Describing the movement of walking to a chair. The bent fingers of the left hand show the sign for "chair"; the index finger of the right hand represents a person moving toward the chair.

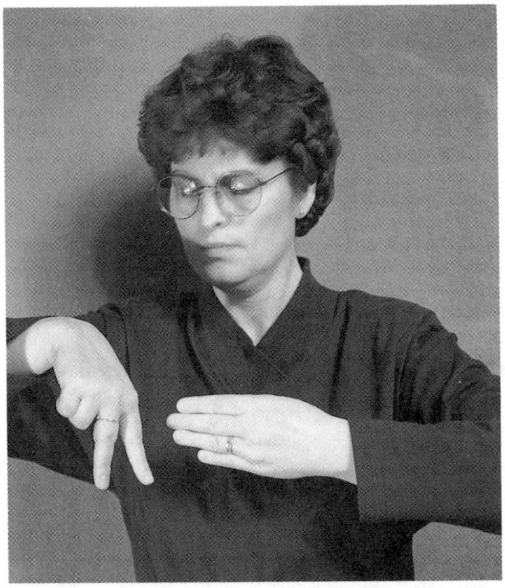

Figure 14. Walking to a wall before squaring off. The person is represented by two fingers pointing down.

To indicate that the surface of the ground is slanted, hold your flat hand horizontal and then slant it the way the surface is tilted. For example, I use my hand to illustrate how streets slope to the gutters, then demonstrate it as we cross a street while the client's hand is on mine. As we start to cross, my hand slowly moves forward and up, then levels off when we reach the middle, and finally slopes forward and down as we approach the other curb. Tilt your hand sideways to show a slope to the side.

Description of a Person's Movement and Position

To indicate a person's movement, use the raised index finger of the active hand to represent the person and move it in the direction or route that you want to explain. If you want to represent movement around or to an object, first name the object (sign, spell, or point to it), represent it with your passive hand, then use the index finger of the active hand to show the "person" moving in relation to where you indicated that the object is (see Figure 13).

If you are emphasizing *how* the person should walk or position himself or herself (for example, "Walk up to the wall and square off against it"), represent the person with two fingers pointing down to represent the legs. The "legs" can walk up to the "wall" (represented with the passive hand) and turn around and square off (see Figure 14).

To say, "Don't step down before you have both feet at the top edge of the stairs," you may first describe the correct way. With the back of your passive hand representing the top of the stairs, have your active hand walk the two-legged "finger fellow" along your passive hand to the "edge" of the "stairs" (that is, to the edge of your hand). Have both "feet" standing squarely on the edge of your hand before one of them "steps" down. To illustrate the incorrect way, have the errant finger fellow walk toward the edge, but before reaching it, reach one "leg" (finger) way out to step down. (Perhaps you can have the finger also lose its balance or trip on the edge to illustrate your point!)

When it is important to emphasize turns, represent the person by the entire flat hand. To show a person walking to a corner, turning, and then crossing, move the flat hand forward (fingers up, little finger toward the front, as illustrated in Figure 15A),

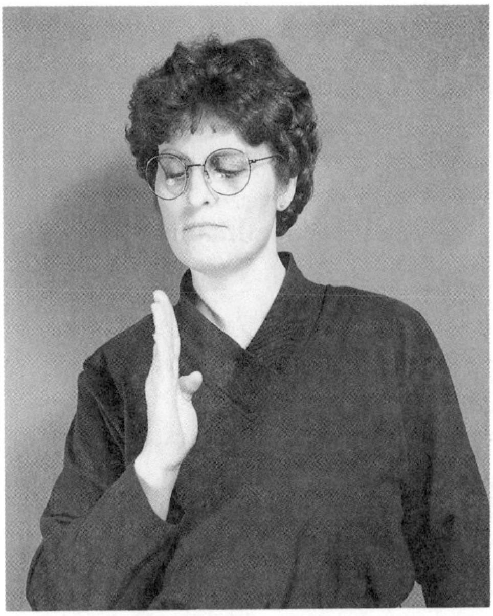

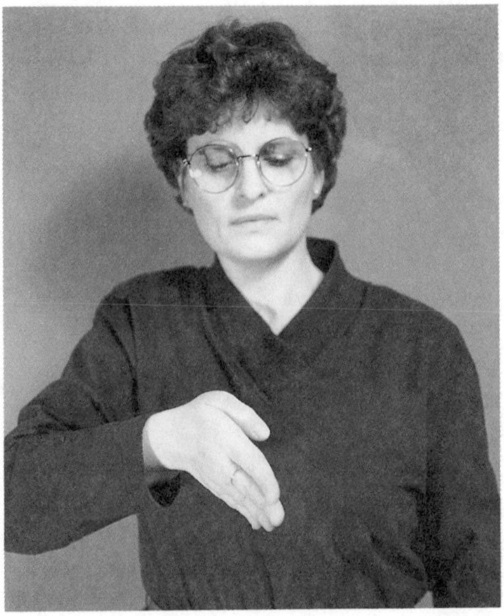

Figures 15A and B. Moving forward and then crossing the street. To emphasize turns, the person is represented by the entire flat hand.

turn the hand, and then "cross" (the hand jumps up and over the imaginary street, starting with fingers pointing up and landing with fingers pointing down, as shown in Figure 15B).

Description of Eye Movements

To tell someone to "look over there," start with your hand in the shape of a V near your eyes, fingers pointing out, and move the hand toward where you want the person to look. To say "Look around the room," scan your V around the room. Eye-scanning techniques and other eye movements can be accurately described by moving the V the way you want the person to move his or her eyes (up and down, side to side, and so forth) (see Figures 16A and B).

Signs for *Cane*

There is no universal sign for a white cane. One sign, which seems to be the most sensible one, is to position the hand as if grasping the handle of the cane, with the forefinger pointing down in the correct position, and pivot the hand from side to side as if moving the cane in the proper arc. However, you must be careful because if this sign is made down too close to the body, it is the sign for a man urinating! Some people put the active hand in the shape of a C on the forearm of the passive hand, but this is the sign for any cane, including a support cane. Other people use the thumb and index finger to trace the shape of the crook and cane (as if moving the finger and thumb along the cane). Again, this sign could

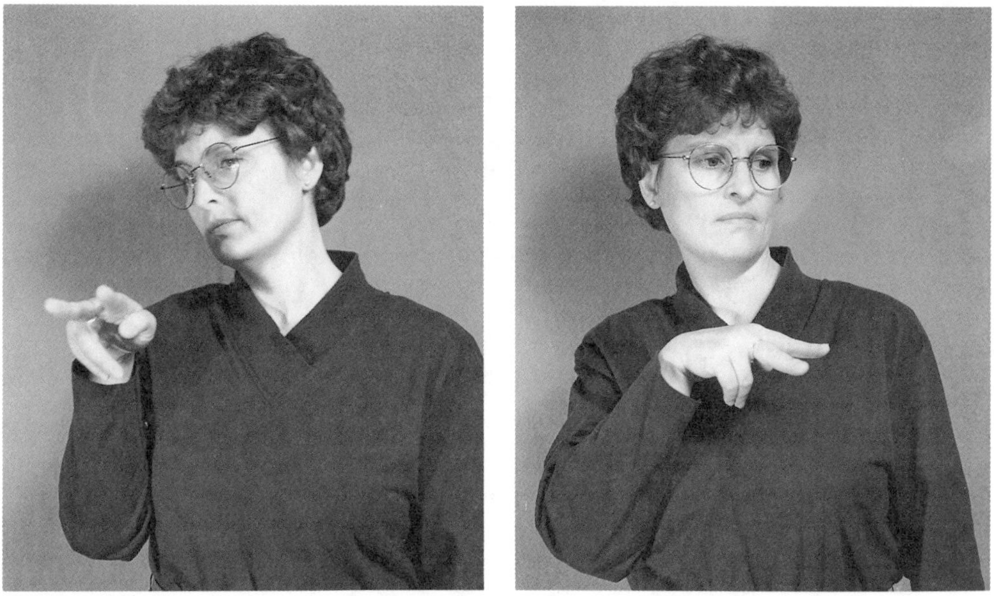

Figures 16A and B. Indicating a look to the right and then to the left. The hand is held in the shape of a V and moved in the direction in which the eyes should move.

signify any cane. When talking with new people, I fingerspell "cane" so I will be understood. When talking with a familiar person, I use whatever sign we have agreed on.

Usually there is no need to sign the word "cane" unless saying something like "Where is your cane?" or "You may need a cane." If you want to say something like, "You need to hold the cane out farther in front of your body," just sign "<should>," then position your hand the way the client is holding the cane, then move it emphatically into the correct position (farther in front of the body). Also, remember that if you are working with a client who is not skilled with English, you should not just translate word for word into signs. He or she may interpret your signs "<hold> <the> <cane> <out>" as meaning literally to grasp the cane outside.

When a client understands what is required for a good cane technique, we often set up signals that we can use as he or she walks. For example, sometimes the client and I decide that tapping on either shoulder means to make the arc wider on that side, tapping the elbow means "out of step," or tapping the hand means the wrist is rotating. If the client can see me while he or she walks, I signify that the arc needs to be wider on the right by holding both hands (palms facing each other) to represent the width of the client's present arc, lifting them, and then emphatically moving the hand that is on the client's right farther to his or her right and lower again. I signify that the client is out of step by holding my arms forward, lifting them slightly and crossing them, and lowering them again.

Description of Cane Movement

The various positions and movements of the cane are easy to describe. Make the index finger of your active hand represent the cane, held at the appropriate angle and moving the way you are trying to describe that the cane moves. You can do this on an imaginary surface in the air or on your passive hand (place the hand horizontally with the palm either up or down) or on the palm of the deaf-blind person. To indicate a cane that is bouncing too high, you can touch your index-finger "cane" on the palm, go way up, and come back down near the fingers. Show the constant-contact cane technique by sliding your fingertip across your flat hand in an arc (see Glossary). The three-point touch technique was described earlier in this chapter (see also Glossary).

CHAPTER 3

COMMUNICATION WITH STRANGERS AND THE PUBLIC

Many people who are deaf-blind need to communicate with persons who have never met an individual with visual and hearing impairments. In such cases, for example, when dealing with the general public, it is usually the deaf-blind person who must initiate and facilitate communication. Frequently, initiating contact and communicating require practice. As Dinsmore (1959, p. 9) stated, "Many [people who are deaf-blind] will need a great deal of help and interpretation if they are to acquire the skill of putting the stranger at ease—of breaking the ice, so to speak."

Some people first need to realize that the method of communication they normally use may not be appropriate with strangers or the public. This is a classic problem for young adults who are congenitally deaf-blind and who use sign language or special communication systems, some of whom expect that strangers will understand their signs or codes. For example, if they learned to request a drink of soda by finding a certain cup and handing it to the teacher, they may later have to learn that at a fast-food restaurant, they need to go to the counter and hand the person a special note or point to a symbol with the word *soda* next to it.

I have found, however, that many people who are adventitiously deaf or blind also do not realize that they must adapt or learn new techniques to communicate with the public. Those who can read notes under good lighting or environmental conditions may not think to bring magnifiers or flashlights to read notes in public. Several people who could understand voice in ideal conditions thought it should not be necessary to use an assistive listening device or other communication method in public, even though background noise usually made it impossible for them to understand others without it. Some people whose visual or hearing impairments were recent had difficulty accepting that they must learn yet another communication method, such as print on palm.

People who are deaf-blind also need to realize that they are responsible for informing others of their communication needs and how others can communicate more clearly with them. The person with sensitive ears and a hearing aid needs to tell others when they are speaking too loudly. The person with restricted visual fields needs to tell those who are using sign language when their signs are too big or too close. The deaf person with limited vision who asks others to write notes needs to inform them that they must write large letters and should provide them with a marker that will write lines thick enough for him or her to see their notes. The person with an interpreter may need to explain to the other person the interpreter's role.

INITIATING COMMUNICATION OR SOLICITING AID

Travelers must be able to solicit aid not only for conventional tasks, such as crossing the street or shopping, but for handling unexpected incidents, such as getting lost, changing a route because of construction, or finding new bus routes. If they are to be safe, independent travelers, even people with minimal language skills must be prepared to handle these situations, perhaps by getting assistance to telephone their home or the police (see "Teaching the Client to Handle an Emergency" in Chapter 9). In some situations, travelers with good communication skills or the ability to use a map can get directions so they can reach their destination themselves. At other times they may need to ask to be guided to their destination or to be assisted to telephone for help to come for them. The instructor can use whatever techniques are appropriate to help deaf-blind people prepare to solicit aid when lost. One effective technique is to provide drop-off lessons (see Glossary) after the client has been thoroughly prepared.

When the person who is deaf-blind needs to solicit aid or communicate, he or she can go where there are likely to be people, such as a bus stop or a street corner or the entrance, service desk, or check-out counter of a store (see Figures 1A–D). Although it is not necessary to find people to get their attention, some deaf-blind people can see or hear well enough to recognize when people are near and others can use an electronic travel aid or vibrotactile device to detect people passing by. When trying to attract attention, mobility instructor William VanBuskirk suggests that travelers should be careful to stand where the public's view of them is not blocked by such obstacles as telephone poles and large displays.

To find out how a deaf-blind person can most effectively solicit aid, David Carrigan and Caryn Spall, both of whom are deaf-blind, agreed to hold up a card to solicit aid to cross streets while Suzanne Jones, Mary Ann Heddleson, and I interviewed people who passed by or who stopped to help (Sauerburger & Jones, 1992). Two different cards were used, to compare the effectiveness of the wording. We found that it is very important for the person who is soliciting aid with a card to appear to want assistance by using gestures or, if wanting to cross a street, by standing at the curb facing the street (see also "Soliciting Aid to Cross Streets" in Chapter 8).

How to Attract Attention

Depending on the person's abilities and the situation, the person who is deaf can use some of the following strategies to get the attention of other people and let them know what he or she needs. If these methods are not effective for certain people, they can brainstorm with their instructors to come up with new ways.

1. Use gestures, such as tapping the cane on the ground while holding it vertically, or appear to be looking for someone to help.
2. Use sound, such as voice or a prerecorded message or a whistle. Although speaking out to ask for assistance can be effective when people's speech is normal, the public often does not realize that they are deaf, even if they tell them. Mobility instructor Michaud (1990, p. 145) wrote that one such person, "Bob, who had perfect speech, often chose to 'turn off his voice' when using the bus. Many times, drivers had called out his stop on the assumption that Bob had heard them." The person needs to be aware of this problem; it may help if he or she signs while talking, since sign language seems to indicate deafness in the same way that a white cane indicates blindness.

   Some travelers get assistance by playing recorded messages. Florence and LaGrow (1989) concluded that a prerecorded message gets people to stop and assist much better than a card, although the subject in their experiment was trying to hand the card to passersby, rather than using the card in the manner that our survey (Sauerburger & Jones, 1992) found to be most effective.

   Some people carry a whistle to blow in an emergency. Rustie Rothstein, a consultant on deaf-blindness, observed that people who blow their whistle for every need should be aware that it can be obnoxious and should try other methods of getting attention.
3. Hold up a note or prewritten card so passersby can read it. The card should be held so it is visible from both the back and the front (at eye level near the shoulder or up above the head). If the card is turned 90 degrees periodically, it is also more likely to be seen by people approaching from any direction.

The card should be easily identifiable to the user (with clipped corners, staples, braille, or holes) and durable (laminated). Some trips will require many cards, thus demanding that they be organized well. For example, a separate card may be needed to cross the street, get the right buses, find the store, and make a purchase. Michaud (1990) reported that some travelers carry their cards in an accordion-style credit-card holder or on a ring, and a few organize them in an index filing box. Rustie Rothstein, a consultant on deaf-blindness, suggested keeping sets of cards needed for each trip organized on a ring (and duplicating cards if they are needed more than once during the trip). If a ring is used, the cards could be designed to be held up on the ring, so the back and front of the cards both show the same message.

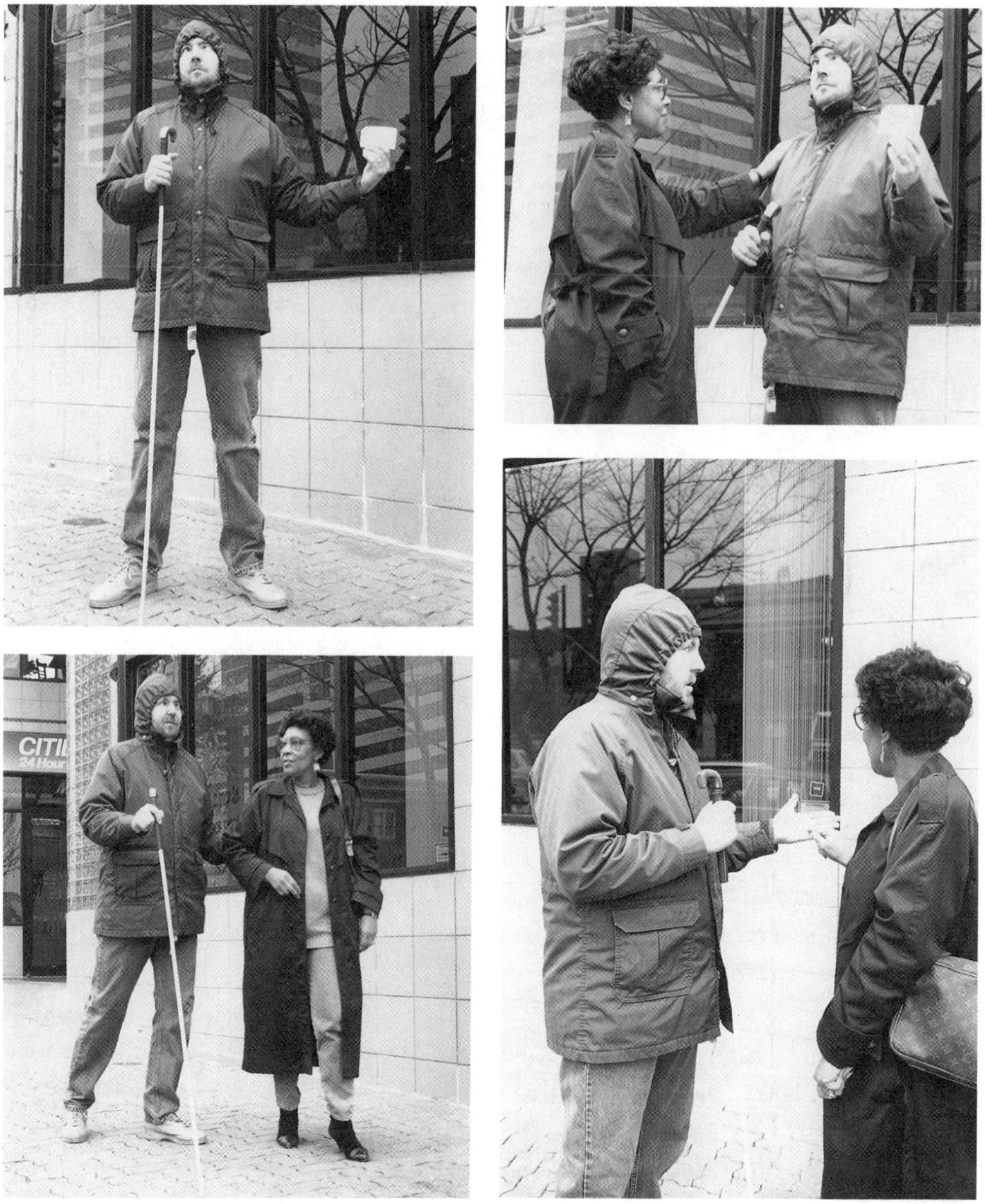

Figures 1 A-D. This deaf-blind man holds up a card requesting information. When tapped, he asks for assistance to find a nearby store and is guided to his destination. His card has also explained how to print on his palm.

Information That Should Be Conveyed

From our interviews (Sauerburger & Jones, 1992) and my experiences, we found that it is important for the traveler to provide information in the following order:

The assistance being requested. When the person's need is not made immediately clear, the public sometimes assumes that he or she is not asking for specific assistance and will walk away without investigating further. Thus, if a card is used, the purpose

("Cross Street") should be in letters large enough to be seen at a distance, printed at or near the top because many people will not read farther than that. In some situations, the words "help me" are needed to clarify that the card is requesting assistance. For example, enlarging those words in the message "Please HELP ME get some INFORMATION" clarifies that the traveler is requesting, not offering, information (see Figure 2).

How others can offer assistance or communicate. If this is not explained promptly and clearly, passersby either assume that the deaf-blind person understands them when they talk or become frustrated or apprehensive when they realize that they cannot communicate with him or her. Then, they either give up or, worse, try to give inappropriate assistance (for example, guide the deaf-blind person where they think he or she wants to go) or call the police to help figure it out.

It is important that the traveler be patient and, if needed, repeat the explanation of how to communicate and, ideally, have several ways of explaining it. Often people do not pay attention or are too surprised to get the explanation the first time.

The person's visual and hearing impairment. It may be best to hold this information for last, since some people are so astonished when they realize that the traveler is deaf and blind that they do not pay attention to the rest of the message. Also, when they read or hear that the traveler is deaf, some people are so bewildered about how to communicate that they walk away.

Preparation of Cards and Recorded Messages

Cards for soliciting aid are available from several sources (see "Communication Books and Cards" in Resources). To be most effective, cards should include information in the order just listed. (See Figure 2 for some examples.) The traveler can make his

Please **HELP ME** get some
INFORMATION
so I can find where I am going.
TAP ME if you can help because I am
DEAF and BLIND.
You can print letters on my palm with
your finger. THANK YOU.

Please **HELP ME** find a
SALESPERSON.
TAP ME if you can help because
I am both **DEAF** AND **BLIND.**
You can **print letters in my palm**
with your **fingertip.** Thank you.

Please help me to
CROSS STREET.
TAP ME if you can help because
I am **DEAF and BLIND**
Thank you!

Figure 2. Some examples of cards used for soliciting aid.

or her own cards; however, if the card appears to be professionally printed, people seem to regard it more respectfully. Neatly typed messages with the key words thickened and enlarged can be copied on two sides of card stock paper (it is a trick to get the copies exactly opposite on each side of the paper). The paper can be cut (perhaps with a clipped corner to indicate the top or bottom), and laminated. Some peel-off lamination or braille sheets can be brailled before they are applied. Use just enough braille to identify the card and position the braille over an empty area (the braille can obscure the print).

A variety of devices are available to generate voice messages either prerecorded (such as the Attention-Getter and Voxcom) or synthesized (see Resources). Several augmentative communication devices have been developed to play recorded messages more conveniently than a tape recorder. Not only can a variety of messages be recorded and played when needed on these solid state electronic devices, they are more reliable than conventional recorders that use magnetic tape. One device is the Attention-Getter, which can play up to 12 messages with a total playing time of 120 seconds. When any one of the buttons is pushed, it plays a certain message; if the button is held down, that message is repeated continuously. The Attention-Getter uses a nine-volt battery and comes with a wrist strap. Messages that will be used outside or in noisy settings should be recorded louder, so that at the regular volume they will play back louder than other messages.

To prevent the message from sounding monotonous when it is repeated, record a pause at the end of each message. Listed next are several suggested messages that follow the same principles for soliciting aid that were found to be effective when using a card. The traveler could play one of the first three messages once or a few times so passersby know what is needed, then play the fourth message so people know how to help. This cycle of messages should be repeated until help is offered. Of course, these are only samples; the actual messages should be worded to meet the needs of the traveler, such as to find a salesperson or a rest room. Some suggested messages are as follows:

"Please help me cross the street." The traveler should face the street he or she wants to cross, and perhaps also point to that street when tapped.

"Please help me catch the right bus." When tapped, the traveler would inform the person of the number of the bus (in voice or with a note). It may also be helpful to hold up a card with the bus number while the message plays.

"I need assistance or information to find my way."

"Tap my shoulder if you can help, because I am deaf and blind" (or "because I cannot hear you.") This message should be played after one of the first three messages.

The deaf-blind person might try each of these methods or a combination of methods to see which is most effective and comfortable for him or her in various situations. Each person is unique, and, as stated by mobility instructor and AFB national program associate Elga Joffee, the characteristics of a particular community can also affect which method would be most efficient in soliciting aid.

PUBLIC RESPONSES

The deaf-blind person can ask the public to respond in various ways, depending on the situation. Some are as follows:

- *Tap the deaf-blind person.* This is one of the simplest ways for the public to respond to indicate their presence or their willingness to help, or to indicate that they understand what is requested.

  Example 1: A woman stands at the curb holding up a card that says, "Please help me cross the street. Tap me if you can help. I am deaf and blind. Thank you." When she is tapped, she smiles and points across the street, then reaches for the other person's arm.

  Example 2: A young man walks into his favorite fast-food restaurant, carrying his set of shopping cards. Because it is difficult for him to learn new things and he has limited language skills, it has taken him many rehearsals to know what to do, but by now he is skilled enough to order his own food. Each card has a square with a texture that is unique, and he has learned to identify what the textures mean. Next to each square is the printed word for that symbol. He approaches the counter and holds out a note that says, "Please tap my hand when you are ready to take my order. I am deaf and blind." When he is tapped, he holds out three cards that say "hamburger," "french fries," and "Sprite" and hands a $5 bill over the counter.
- *Write or spell to the deaf-blind person.* People who are deaf-blind may ask the other person to spell out a message in one of several ways, such as to use a finger to print letters on their palm, give the person paper and a marker thick enough for them to read and ask the person to write a note, or have the person type into their Teletouch machine.

  Example: A man enters a dry cleaner, finds the counter, and writes a note to the saleswoman that says, "Please tell me when these clothes can be ready. You can print on my palm with your finger. I am deaf and blind." The saleswoman looks at the note and tells the man that the clothes can be ready by Wednesday. Realizing that the saleswoman did not understand, the man demonstrates to her how to print on his palm, holds out his hand, and gestures for the saleswoman to print on the palm. The saleswoman pauses for a moment, then prints, "The clothes can be ready Wednesday."
- *Speak to the deaf-blind person.* The deaf-blind person may need to explain to the public how they should speak so he or she can understand. For example, people may be asked to talk in a normal voice close to the ear, to speak into the traveler's microphone, or to stand in or under good lighting so the traveler can lipread.

Example: A blind traveler enters a hair-styling salon and says, "Can someone help me, please?" The receptionist responds, and the traveler holds out a microphone while saying, "I'd like to know if I can get my hair cut this afternoon. Please speak into this microphone using a normal tone of voice because I can't hear well."

- *Signal yes or no.* The deaf-blind person may ask others to tap once for yes and twice for no or vice versa; three times for "Please repeat"; and four times for "I don't know." Another signal if the person can see well enough is to nod the head yes or no.

  Example: A bus pulls up to a stop where a woman with a white cane stands waiting. She gets on the bus and hands the driver a note that says, "Is this the 37 bus? Please tap me twice if yes, once if no. I am deaf and can't see well." She holds her hand out, and the driver taps twice. She puts her money in the coin box, hands the driver a note with instructions to let her know when the bus arrives at her stop, and a passenger helps her find an empty seat.

Since no method is guaranteed to be effective for communicating with every person whom the deaf-blind person may encounter, it may help to realize that it is not always his or her fault when communication breaks down or when the other person acts strangely. If the communication goes awry a few times while you are present unobtrusively, it can become less mystifying to the deaf-blind person to find out whatever you were able to observe or discover about the encounter.

To make the response understandable to a person with limited language skills or to save time in a hectic situation, the deaf-blind person may ask the public to respond in a structured and specific way. This response can be designed to fit the situation and the traveler's skills, such as yes-no answers, or specific responses to particular instructions.

For example, a young deaf client who is developmentally disabled and has good central vision went to buy an item. He could write notes and could read and understand simple written sentences. When he first went to a store and handed the clerk a note asking for an item, the clerk wrote back, "We carry that item, but it won't be here until the truck arrives Monday." Needless to say, the client did not understand, smiled, and walked up and down the aisles for 20 minutes looking for the item until I intervened.

To make sure the clerk's response would be understood by the client, we developed a checklist for him to bring to the store, with several choices for the clerk to check. The client learned ahead of time what each choice meant, so he could know what the clerk's response indicated. His note said,

> I am deaf and can't see well. I would like to buy a ————. Please check one of the following:
>
> 1. — We have the item. I will get it for you. It costs ————.
> 2. — We don't carry that item.
> 3. — We carry that item but don't have it right now. We should have it by ————.

There are countless ways that the response of the public or shopkeeper can be structured for people whose language skills are limited. Structuring the public's response can also simplify the situation or facilitate the communication when the situation is hectic. For example, a deaf client with restricted visual fields but good central vision did not know the bus stop nearest to her destination. Before her trip, she drew a simple map to show to the driver and a note that said, "Please point on this map where the bus can let me off near 20th Street and Maple. I am deaf and visually impaired. Thank you." This strategy worked well, and the driver pointed to 20th and Maple on the map.

The principle of simplifying the situation by structuring the response can be useful. People who are unsure which way they are facing can use their preferred communication method to ask another person to indicate which way is downtown or such-and-such a street by pointing. If they cannot see the other person, they can ask if they can feel the other person's hand pointing or ask the other person to turn them to face the right direction. When looking for the entrance to a nearby store or the doctor's office in a medical building, for example, they can ask someone to guide them. On the rapid transit system, travelers who are not sure which of their fare cards has enough funds remaining to get to their destination can ask the station attendant to look at the cards and tap the correct card.

TEACHING SUCCESSFUL COMMUNICATION

When teaching people to communicate with the public, the instructor might start with structured situations (for which the communication is simple and predictable) and progress to increasingly unstructured situations (for which it is less predictable and requires a lot of thinking and strategies). For example, before they try to solicit information to find an unfamiliar store or get reoriented, deaf-blind people should have experience communicating effectively with strangers. One suggested progression of situations may be to practice communicating to

- solicit aid to cross streets;
- shop in small stores (especially places like dry cleaners, where the person knows in advance what kinds of information will be requested);
- call for bus information;
- buy something at fast-food restaurants;
- shop in a large department store;
- use a bus;
- solicit aid to get to an unfamiliar destination; or
- solicit assistance to figure out where he or she is when lost.

The use of a bus is not near the beginning of the list because people first need to be comfortable communicating with the public and be experienced in coping when things go wrong. Bus drivers have little time to try to understand travelers, and it can be a frustrating and negative experience for both unless the deaf-blind person is prepared.

Based partly on Michaud's (1990) suggestions and partly on my experience, the following are some factors that seem to contribute to acquiring the communication skills needed for the greatest amount of independent travel:

1. The person is motivated to be independent and to communicate with the public.
2. The person is able to inform the public how to communicate with him or her, help them become comfortable enough to try it, repeat the explanation as needed, and remain patient and calm when things do not go well.
3. The person can use several methods of communication and is flexible enough to adapt to the situation with an appropriate method.
4. The person is organized and keeps any equipment or materials needed for communication readily accessible, so the interaction can start and proceed smoothly.
5. The person can communicate spontaneously and is not limited to communications (such as prewritten notes) that must be prepared ahead of time.
6. The person can understand English (spelled or verbal).

Deaf-blind people who do not have all (or any) of these characteristics may still be able to communicate with the public to some degree. However, they should develop as many of these characteristics as is practical so they can achieve their potential for independent travel.

INTERPRETING FOR THE PUBLIC

People sometimes approach us when a deaf-blind person and I are working together in public. This is a great opportunity for the person to interact with other people, either

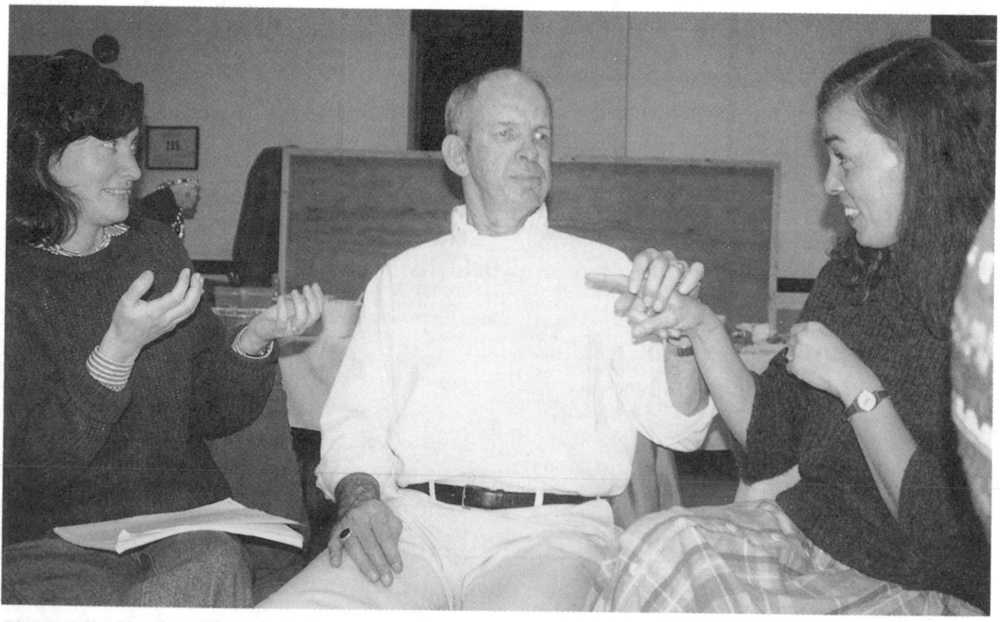

Figure 3. As the woman on the left talks, this deaf-blind man knows who is speaking because his interpreter first points to the person before translating what is being said.

directly or through an interpreter. Because many people who are deaf or deaf-blind are accustomed to people speaking for them, some refrain from expressing themselves and depend on the service provider or family member to do it for them. To avoid this situation, I explain ahead of time that when the opportunity presents itself, I will step out of the role of instructor and become an impartial interpreter (see "Establishing Roles" in Chapter 1).

We also establish (and practice, if necessary) how the deaf-blind person will know who is speaking. I usually indicate this fact by pointing to whomever is speaking (including myself) before I interpret what that person is saying. If I am spelling out words (such as with fingerspelling or Teletouch), I spell out the name of the speaker ("bus driver says. . ." or "Shirley says. . ."). (See Figure 3.)

People tend to talk not with a blind person or a deaf person, but with whomever is with that person. When the person is both deaf and blind and is with a service provider, you can imagine how difficult it is for people to realize that they should speak directly to that person. The deaf-blind person should be made aware (through accurate interpreting) that this is happening, and correct it if he or she wishes (see "Establishing Roles" in Chapter 1).

I found that this problem can usually be avoided if I say, "A man [or woman or salesperson or policeman] has approached us. Do you want me to interpret?" I say it in a voice loud enough for the other person to hear, but I speak to (and keep my eyes on) the deaf-blind person and interpret what I am saying. During the conversation, I avoid eye contact with the other person, usually looking at the deaf-blind person or down at the floor. Most people get the hint and speak to the deaf-blind person or, if they want to talk to me, they realize that I am interpreting what we are saying. However, Leslie Leopold, who coordinates services for deaf-blind people, noted that the person should choose whether to reveal to the stranger that he or she is deaf and should be encouraged to assert his or her own interpreting needs, rather than have the worker say, "Shall I interpret for you?" Thus, you may explain to the deaf-blind person the implications of this situation ahead of time and discuss how he or she wants it to be handled.

CHAPTER 4

INTERACTION WITH THE PUBLIC

People who are deaf-blind can interact independently with the public to do almost anything—shop, go to work, visit a physician, find an address or get directions, take a bus or taxi, and so on. However, what often typifies interaction undertaken without preparation and awareness can be summed up in one word: misunderstanding. The public usually does not understand that the person has a hearing impairment as well as a visual impairment. If they realize that the person is deaf, they usually do not know how they can communicate or interact with him or her and often feel awkward or bewildered when they first try it. Many are also incredulous that a person who is deaf and blind can travel independently in the community.

The failure of the public to understand the situation is often compounded by the deaf-blind person's failure to recognize that the public is bewildered. Klara Johnson (1992), who is deaf-blind, recounted the following experience about when she realized for the first time that strangers do not know how to approach her: When her friend was late to pick her up at a train station, she "became more and more concerned, for I could not see or hear what was going on around me. Finally I called out, 'Is anyone there?' Nothing happened, so I called again. Still nothing happened. People may well have been there, but if so, they did not know what to do to help me—for all I know, they may have spoken to me, even offered help.

"When I realized this, I called out again, 'I am deaf and blind, you must touch me for me to know you are there.' And someone did touch my hand; someone did reach out to me because I was able to show them how. I was no longer alone, no longer afraid. My friend arrived shortly thereafter, but the lesson I had learned remained with me."

Many people who are deaf-blind, regardless of their experience, intelligence, or visual and hearing impairments, assume that the other person in a situation knows they are deaf or that the other person will know how to communicate with them without being told (or after being told only once). At first, I did not know why people did not respond appropriately after my clients had clearly told them that they were deaf and explained how to communicate with them. Like my clients, I thought that perhaps they were deliberately being inconsiderate or that they preferred not to interact with a person who is deaf-blind. Only when I spoke with these people afterward did I realize they were not responding because they had not grasped the deaf-blind person's first explanation (see "The Story of John"). To find out more about this phenomenon, Suzanne Jones, Mary Ann Heddleson, and I interviewed dozens of people who passed by or helped a deaf-blind person who was displaying an explanatory card (Sauerburger & Jones, 1992). We learned that regardless of what was written on the card, many people (even some of those who helped) did not realize that the person was deaf or did not know how to interact with the person.

THE STORY OF JOHN

It was by teaching mobility to an intrepid man named John that I was able to learn answers to some of the mysteries of the public's reaction to deaf-blind people. While John traveled during his mobility lessons, I observed him telling other people that he is deaf and that they should print their message on his palm with their finger. These people all seemed kind and eager to help, yet for several weeks he explained how to communicate numerous times without a single person trying to print on his palm or communicate in any way except to continue to talk or gesture and point. Perplexed, I was determined to find out why they were unable or unwilling to communicate with him as he asked.

One day, a man helped John cross the street and walked with him for part of the next block. I saw that, as usual, John had tried to show him how to communicate. As usual, the man persisted in talking and asking him questions that John could not hear. After he left John, the man walked past me, and I asked him, "Will that blind man be all right?" The man stopped and said, "You know, come to think of it, he might be deaf. His card said he was deaf, and his answers to all my questions weren't appropriate. Let me go and see." He went back to John and yelled, "Are you deaf?" John walked into him and then around him, totally unaware that anyone was there. The man came back, and I could see he was astonished. He was mumbling to himself, "My god! Deaf *and* blind! If I write to him, he won't see it, and he can't hear me! How can I talk to him?"

I asked if "the blind man" had shown him how to print on his palm (I knew that John had), but he said no. I then told him how it is done, demonstrating it on my palm. He looked at me but appeared to be still dumbfounded, and I could see he was not paying attention. So I showed him the printing on his own palm. His eyes lit up, and he ran to catch up with John, eager to try this method.

John was glad to have someone finally communicate with him, and they began a conversation. The man then wrote in John's palm, "You can write in my palm." At first John looked puzzled, then he nodded and wrote "Are you deaf, too?" The man, realizing

(continued on next page)

On the basis of these discussions and interviews with the public, it seems that there are various reasons why many people do not grasp the deaf-blind person's explanations. Some of them just are not paying attention or are preoccupied. Others are attentive, but when they realize the person is deaf-blind they are so shocked they are unable to think clearly or understand the explanation. Still others are cognizant, but they find it so inconceivable that a person who is deaf-blind could be traveling independently that they fail to realize that the person they are with indeed has both a hearing and a visual impairment. When they realize that the person is blind or visually impaired, they often do not consider that the person could be deaf as well.

AWARENESS OF THE PUBLIC'S INCOGNIZANCE

The person who is deaf-blind needs to realize that even when the situation is carefully explained, the public sometimes does not grasp that he or she is deaf-blind or

that since he could hear and understand John, John did not have to print in his hand, laughed at his own mistake. Nevertheless, even after he made sure John knew where he was and was going the right way, the man flagged down a policeman to keep an eye on John.

We had many experiences like this in subsequent lessons, where I made the effort to talk with people after John's encounter with them (usually without them knowing that I was with John). Once I had just finished talking with John and was standing on the sidewalk a few feet away when a well-dressed, intelligent-looking man approached John to help him cross the street. He apparently wanted to say something to John. John clearly and slowly explained and demonstrated to the man how to print on his palm and held his hand out for the man to print on. The man watched the explanation carefully, but then just guided John across the street without trying to print on his palm. I assumed that the man had changed his mind and did not want to talk, so I was surprised when he returned to ask me how to communicate with John. He apparently had been too dumbfounded to grasp it when John himself explained. I suggested we go and ask John to explain again, which we did. This time the man understood, and they enjoyed a pleasant conversation.

John (like many other people who are deaf-blind) had often assumed that other people were not communicating with him because they were stupid, or mean, or just did not want to talk with a person who is deaf-blind. I sometimes assumed the same things, but I have now talked with enough people to know that they usually wanted to talk or to help but did not know how to do so.

Now that he knows why many people do not respond to him, John tries to put people at ease and patiently and clearly repeats his explanation of how to communicate until they finally get it. Other deaf-blind people have been equally surprised to learn that most strangers sincerely want to help but cannot comprehend the situation. This realization has helped them to be more patient with the public and to persist until they establish communication.

Adapted from Dona Sauerburger, "Moving Right Along: Orientation & Mobility for Deaf-Blind Persons," *Deaf-Blind American*, December 1988, pp. 11–15.

does not understand how to communicate. The deaf-blind person sometimes needs to explain the situation several times in different ways until people respond as expected. He or she also needs to realize that when people seem to act inappropriately, they are usually not being intentionally rude, but are unaware that the person is deaf or do not know how to communicate, regardless of how they were informed.

Some deaf-blind people may assume that the public is aware of their deafness because when they were sighted, people usually recognized that they were deaf. Now that they are both visually impaired and deaf, they need to realize that the public has a hard time recognizing or accepting that someone who uses a white cane may also be deaf. Other deaf-blind people believe that the public is too competent to be so ignorant. One woman was reluctant to explain to others how to communicate with her through the interpreter because she thought that hearing people are "clever" and already know how to do so. She did not realize that most people know little about deafness and less about interpreters and that they need her help to understand the interpreter's role and feel comfortable interacting with her.

THE STORY OF KATHY

Kathy had been living independently for several years and had impaired vision and hearing since birth. However, when she lost more of her vision and some of her physical stamina, she moved to an assisted-living apartment and stopped traveling independently. A year later, she got an electric scooter and requested O&M lessons. Her speech was understandable, and I communicated with her by speaking clearly while signing close to her.

Kathy wanted to be able to go to the store herself again. She said she already knew how to communicate, so I did not review communication procedures. She brought a tablet of paper and a wide-tipped marker to the area in front of her building where the shuttle bus takes residents to the store. However, although she knew effective communication techniques, she apparently did not know how to assess the situation with strangers and come up with the most effective communication technique, inform them of her needs, and patiently repeat the explanation if they failed to respond.

We waited for the bus with other residents, some of whom were in wheelchairs. When a bus arrived, Kathy asked the others if this was the bus that went to the store. She could not hear their answers, so she told them she was deaf and asked them again. They answered more loudly, but she still could not understand.

I explained to Kathy that simply telling others that she is deaf does not help them know how to communicate with her. When she could not think of how they could respond so she could understand them, I gave her several suggestions. She chose to ask them to nod their heads yes if the bus went to the store and no if it did not. They shook their heads no. She then asked them when her bus would arrive, but again she could not understand their answers. Eventually, she handed them her paper and marker and asked them to write the answer. This effort was successful.

(continued on next page)

People who are deaf-blind can be naive about communicating with the public even though they are capable and experienced (see "The Story of Kathy"). Some people who are deaf-blind believe they have a right to expect others to understand their needs and, as one person put it, to "meet me halfway." They are probably right; it is not fair that they should have to explain everything so many times. However, if they want to interact with others—for information, to get a job, to get help to cross the street, to buy something, or to make new friends—they will usually have to do more than their share to make the interaction go smoothly.

SUCCESSFUL INTERACTIONS

If the deaf-blind person is prepared with communication methods that the public can understand and recognizes that others usually need clear, careful explanations of how to interact, it is likely that the interactions will go well (see, for example, Figures 1A and B). A lot of patience and a warm sense of humor go a long way, too. Most important, the person who is deaf-blind needs to monitor how others are reacting and be persistent.

When another bus pulled up to the apartment building, the other people pointed to the bus and nodded yes. The driver got out and asked Kathy and several others if they could get out of their wheelchairs to transfer to the bus seat. Kathy could not understand him, but again she did not instruct him how to communicate. The driver started to load the other passengers onto the lift, and I surreptitiously signed to Kathy that she should tell him how to communicate. When the driver approached her, Kathy gave him the paper and marker, explained that she is deaf, and asked the driver to write what he was trying to say. The driver wrote, "Can you get out of the scooter?" Kathy answered yes.

After the driver loaded another passenger, he came back and verbally asked Kathy to back her scooter onto the lift. Evidently the driver, as do many other people, needed more than one explanation of how to communicate. Kathy looked perplexed, but she did not hand the driver the paper or remind him to write. The driver then tried in vain to steer her scooter onto the lift, ran over his toe, and finally gave up. He said he was afraid to take Kathy because he could not communicate with her. He left her at the bus stop, puzzled and perplexed.

Although this was a frustrating experience, after Kathy was told what had happened, she realized what she needed to do. At our next session, we went to a shopping mall, where she tentatively began to inform others how to communicate with her and to repeat the explanation patiently, if necessary. These experiences were successful, and her communication skills became excellent. As soon as she noticed someone talking to her or whenever she approached people for assistance, she handed them her pen and tablet and asked them to write their message in large letters, explaining that she is deaf and cannot see well. She said she loved to go shopping.

If the other person does not respond or responds inappropriately, the person who is deaf-blind needs to try to figure out the cause of the other person's reaction and give additional explanations or try another approach until there is an appropriate response. For example, Jack Wright, who is deaf-blind, entered a store and held up a card that said, "I need to find a salesperson. I am deaf and blind, so please tap me if you can help. You can print letters on my palm with your finger." He occasionally tapped his cane to draw attention, but when he got no response, he searched for and found a counter. There he bumped into a customer and showed the card again. The customer tried to help by pointing across the counter where a salesperson was. Finally, a saleslady approached and touched him and said, "May I help you?" Jack pointed several times to the card, hoping she would read how to print on his palm. She said, "Yes, I *am* a salesperson! How can I help you?" After perceiving no response but verifying that she was still there, Jack put the card away and demonstrated how to print on his palm. That technique did not work either (she thought he was asking for a pen). He then took out his pad and pen and wrote a note that said what he wanted to buy and that asked her to answer by printing on his palm. She finally did so, and he was able to make his purchase. Jack was successful because he was patient, persistent, and skilled in several methods of expressive communication with the public (use of cards, gestures, demonstrations, and writing notes). In cases in which salespeople do not respond, the deaf-blind person might try telling the salesperson how to signal that he or she is too busy to help right away. For example, the shopper could write or say, "If I need to wait a few minutes for assistance, please tap my hand twice" (see Chapter 3 for further ideas).

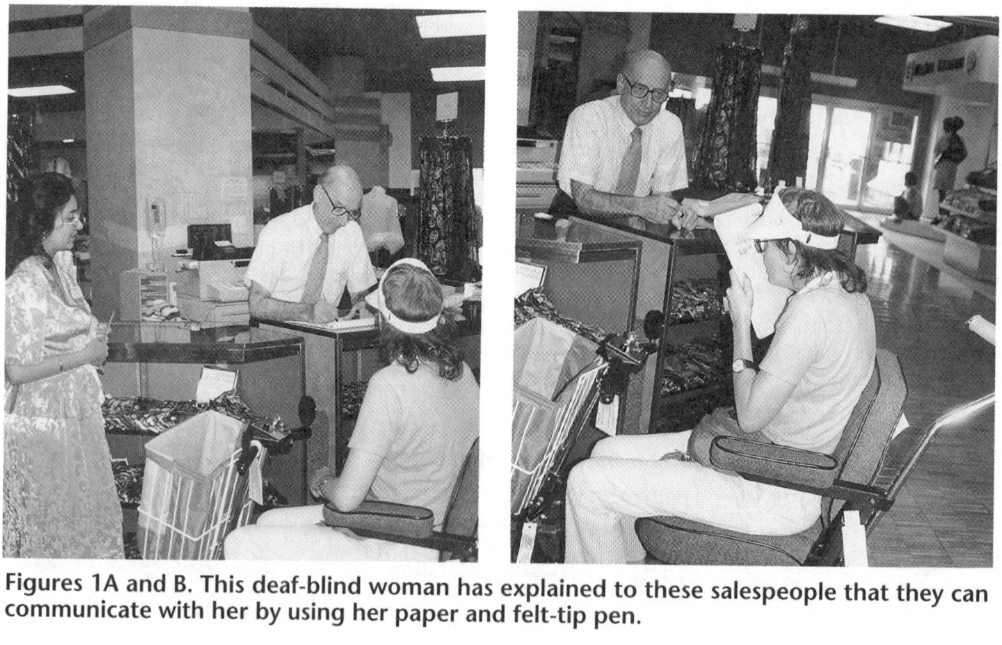

Figures 1A and B. This deaf-blind woman has explained to these salespeople that they can communicate with her by using her paper and felt-tip pen.

UNDERSTANDING THE PUBLIC'S REACTION

When people cannot ascertain exactly what others are doing or why, they sometimes assume the worst. Occasionally, newly blinded people tell me they think everyone is watching them, when no one is paying any attention. Sometimes deaf people suspect that others may be talking about them. It has been said that the "reality checker" of blind or deaf people is impaired—that they cannot verify exactly what is happening around them. The reality checker of people whose vision and hearing are both impaired, however, is even more damaged.

Dorothy Stiefel, who is hearing impaired and losing her vision, wrote (1991, pp. 50, 53, 54), "Everyone at one time or another. . . will. . .misjudge or misinterpret what is observed, but. . .I am misinterpreting much more often what I perceive to be happening around me. . . . I try to be alert to signs of paranoia. . . . Losing the ability to make valid, perceptive judgments about what I have seen and/or heard makes me feel very vulnerable. Do I continue to interact normally and risk the emotional consequences of unsuitable behavior, or should I be more reticent, subdued, and avoid active socialization?"

When people have numerous disconcerting experiences, such as those discussed next, without understanding why people behaved as they did, it is easy for them to become exasperated and distrustful of the public:

> A young deaf woman with a severely restricted visual field was outgoing and trusting. During her mobility lesson, she went to the manager's office at her grocery store with a note that said, "Please tell me where the raisins are located." The staff told her, but she could not understand them. They tried several ways to help, finally motioning for her to follow one of them. She started to follow, but soon lost him. She returned to where she and I had agreed to meet. She was almost in tears, saying in sign language, "They were so *mean* to me! Who do they hate me?" I was surprised at her reaction and explained what really happened. This explanation consoled her greatly because she had not realized they were trying hard to help. The next time, her note asked them to write the directions or aisle number for her.

> A deaf man with a visual impairment was riding a bus, sitting next to a helpful woman. When he was ready to get off, he turned to her and said "thank you" as politely as he could in both sign language and voice. The lady suddenly yelled at him and hit him with her purse. Fortunately, his mobility instructor saw it happen and explained to him that the lady yelled, "Don't you dare blow kisses to me!"

When a person seems to act strangely, the deaf-blind person needs to consider what the cause may have been. Often, as happened in the first example, the person did not know how to communicate (or that the person was deaf and blind), even if the person who is deaf-blind explained how to do so. Occasionally, as in the second example, it is a coincidental misunderstanding. Robert J. Smithdas, who is deaf-blind, recalls holding out a note to ask for assistance from a man who ignored him and then finding out that the man was blind. Other travelers have verbally asked for assistance from people who are deaf and have handed notes to people who could not respond because they were illiterate or did not speak English. If people who are deaf-blind have no experience from which to draw possible rationales, they may jump to the only conclusion they can think of—that the other person hates disabled people or is purposely being rude.

Role of the Instructor

The deaf-blind person may understand the public's behavior better if the instructor discusses what has been explained in this chapter. In addition, he or she needs objective feedback about his or her efforts to interact with the public. Therefore, once the deaf-blind person has learned the skills needed to travel independently in business areas and communicate with the public, the instructor should step back and observe unobtrusively as the person tries these new skills. The instructor later reports to the person whatever happened: whether people stopped and stared, turned away, tried unsuccessfully to communicate with him or her, admired what the person was accomplishing, seemed pleased to be able to help, or acted impatient or disgusted.

Try to describe this behavior objectively. For example, rather than say, "The store manager was really nervous," explain that "her hands were trembling and she looked away from you." Let the person who is deaf-blind form his or her own impression of the meaning of the other person's comments, behavior, facial expressions, and body language.

Often, when I am puzzled about why some people behaved as they did, I will approach them without letting them know I am associated with the deaf-blind person and innocently ask what happened. By doing so, I learn that usually the people behaved as they did because they did not understand the situation, even though the client explained it to them clearly. Their answers are usually revealing, and I share that information with the client. It takes time to give deaf-blind people this information, especially if the communication method is slow, but it is worth the effort if clients begin to have a more realistic understanding of their world and their effect on other people. When traveling alone after training, they are more likely to understand the seemingly incomprehensible way people act if the instructor took the time during training to help clarify it.

Welsh (1980, p. 238) described this role of the instructor with any visually impaired client: "As the lessons progress, the mobility specialist retreats farther and farther from the client, increasing the chances that others will approach him and offer help or otherwise interact. As the client gets experience by dealing with people as well as evaluative feedback from the specialist about these interactions, some of [the client's] anxieties can be overcome." The need for unobtrusive observation and evaluative feedback is even greater for blind clients who cannot hear.

Honest Feedback

When describing to deaf-blind people what you observed about their interaction with the public, you should *not* try to smooth over or rationalize your comments—the person who is deaf-blind needs and deserves honesty. However, it is sometimes difficult to be honest. Years ago, I was teaching a polite woman who is deaf-blind. As we were leaving a fast food establishment that she had just successfully found during her lesson, the manager approached me and said in a foreign accent, "We don't want any of that kind in here. Do not let her come back again." I did not have the heart to interpret what he said, but realize now that I should have been honest, no matter how difficult it would have been.

I no longer shield people from harsh realities. If I had known then what I know now, when the manager approached me I would have immediately communicated to the woman (while voicing so the manager could hear), "The manager is speaking to us. Do you want me to interpret?" The manager could then have conveyed his message to her directly, and she would have had an opportunity to face him and respond. If she had not been with me when he approached, I would have suggested that I come back later with her and interpret while he told her his message himself. In any case, I would have told her what happened.

Being cut off from much of the world is probably the most devastating result of deaf-blindness, and it is through the eyes and ears of others that deaf-blind people can try to gain an understanding of what may seem to them (and sometimes to us) to be an irrational world. It is only when we are honest that people who are deaf-blind can learn to trust us to tell them what is really happening.

When the Instructor Should Step In

After the deaf-blind person has learned how to communicate skillfully with strangers and is prepared for their possible reactions, he or she is ready to interact with the public. When the situation becomes awkward, you must judge whether the client would benefit more from intervention and immediate feedback or from trying to cope with the situation. It is important to give deaf-blind people the opportunity to cope independently with circumstances and to provide them with feedback later. However, in some cases the client may need immediate feedback or reminders of what to do in a situation.

It is also important to remember that if the instructor allows the client to have negative experiences before he or she is ready, the client may be too frustrated and discouraged to continue to learn to interact with the public. However, some instructors may be overly concerned about this possibility and think the deaf-blind person needs to be sheltered from all difficulties and disappointments. This unrealistic expectation may make us interfere when we should let the client experience the aggravations that real life offers everyone. We need to realize that even with extensive preparation and extreme competence, interactions will not always go smoothly. Clients must learn to deal with the frustration that can result when even their best efforts are not enough. In addition, some clients need to experience what can happen when the public does not know what to do, so they can fully appreciate the need to inform the public how to communicate. It is also important to remember that many people learn best from their own mistakes. If the instructor steps in whenever things become awkward, the client may take longer to learn how to avoid the awkwardness or may never learn how to deal with embarrassment or frustration.

When I first started teaching people who are deaf-blind, I found it difficult to refrain from making everything go smoothly during the client's interaction with other people. I was tempted to step forward and explain to the bewildered public how to communicate with my client when they could not understand his or her explanations. At other times I wanted to remind clients when they forgot to inform the public how to communicate with them.

I was tempted to interfere partly because I felt responsible for making everything go smoothly (which I have already explained is impossible). At other times, however, I was embarrassed and anxious because I thought that people might realize that I was the instructor and think that I should help. Most mobility instructors have experienced this embarrassment to a lesser degree when working with hearing blind clients. What instructor has not been glared or yelled at by drivers or pedestrians who see him or her standing on the corner and not helping "that poor blind person" standing nearby? Yet competent mobility instructors do not let that embarrassment discourage them from allowing their blind clients to be as independent as possible. This is just as true with the deaf-blind client who is learning to interact with the public. When things become awkward, the instructor will have to exercise good judgment to determine whether the client will learn more by being allowed to try to figure things out alone or by having the instructor step in and become involved.

The first time that the public was baffled about a client and started to call the police, I stepped in immediately and explained the situation. Now, I try to prepare the deaf-blind person to expect such circumstances. If people call the police, I let the situation unfold as it would have happened if I were not there. It is better for the client to experience it when I can observe and tell him or her afterwards what happened.

When the police showed up after such a call, their intervention was not unpleasant. One who had been called by a bewildered salesperson placed the client's hand on his badge and gun, the client showed him how to communicate, and the two of them went off to finish the shopping, having a pleasant conversation (the client wrote notes on paper, and the policeman wrote back on his palm). Another policeman who had been called by a concerned citizen observed the client briefly and drove off, realizing that the client was all right. One man called the police because he got no answer when he repeatedly offered to help my client (who was obviously lost). I was with the client when the policeman arrived and asked us if everything was all right. I interpreted, to allow the client to respond and handle the situation himself. The client was pleased with all the attention and told the story to all his friends.

However, deaf-blind people have told me about situations in which the police arrested them because of misunderstandings. One deaf visually impaired man walked through a metal detector and did not stop when they said several times to halt. He was thrown to the floor and handcuffed, unable to explain that he was deaf. Intervention from an instructor may not have helped in this situation; the deaf-blind man's friend had arrived to meet him, but he was not able to convince the police that the man was deaf or prevent him from being taken to jail.

Obviously, it is difficult to remain out of the situation if the public realizes that an instructor is nearby because people invariably ignore the deaf-blind person and attempt to have the instructor intercede with the client for them (sometimes becoming angry when the instructor will not cooperate). If possible, I deny that I am with the client (technically, I am not "with" him or her) or I explain that I must remain neutral. I then leave if the client is not in danger. I avoid explaining that the person is deaf; he or she needs to know whether the public understands it without my telling them.

To avoid being noticed, the instructor can behave and dress inconspicuously. Although I have not tried this during a lesson, I have noticed, while videotaping people who were wearing small microphones, that I could be far away from them and still hear what was going on through their microphones. Perhaps using a microphone (inconspicuously clipped to the deaf-blind person's shirt), the instructor could remain out of sight or at a distance while observing what was happening around the deaf-blind person. The set can be purchased in such places as Radio Shack and photography-supply stores, and it can be used unobtrusively without the camera.

Ways of Coping with the Public

Effective travelers who are deaf-blind are keenly aware of and often mention the importance of being presentable and gracious whenever they are in public, since they never know when a potential helper may be observing. They also let the public know that their help is appreciated.

Sometimes deaf-blind travelers are overwhelmed by the inability of the public to realize that they are capable and can travel independently in the community. A few even question their own abilities and rights in view of the negative or patronizing attitudes of some people. It sometimes helps when I inform them that I observed the same reaction to independent blind travelers 20 years ago, when most people had never seen a blind person traveling alone. Blind travelers are commonplace now, but most people have never seen a deaf-blind traveler before. They often respect the rights and recognize the capabilities of blind people but cannot yet imagine it possible that people who are deaf-blind can get around independently. This attitude can be frustrating to deaf-blind people, and they have every right to be indignant, but if they realize that they are doing something that the public finds amazing, it can be a source of great pride and satisfaction.

Deaf-blind people who find it difficult to cope with the frustration of dealing with the public may also benefit from talking about it with other travelers who are deaf-blind or who have other disabilities. Many people who are deaf-blind are surprised to find out that they are not the only ones who experience disbelief or condescension from the public; most successful travelers with disabilities, including hearing travelers who are blind or who use wheelchairs, also experience it to some degree.

ESTABLISHING GUIDELINES FOR LESSONS IN PUBLIC

The instructor and client need to be prepared for problems that arise during lessons in public. One such problem is that when a stranger approaches, the client sometimes thinks it is the instructor. One night, my client, who had a narrow field of vision, got into a young couple's car with them, thinking that the woman was me, and was driven to her destination. Another client, also with a narrow field of vision, arrived at the top of the escalators when exiting the public transit system into bright sunlight and allowed a man to lead her back down the escalators, thinking that the man was me. Therefore, you must establish a signal to identify yourself so the client knows when you, not a stranger, is approaching.

Another problem is that some clients are not accustomed to communicating with others independently. They let the public control the conversation, standing until the other person is done, sometimes answering personal questions. Clients should be encouraged to enjoy communicating with others, but they also need to realize that if they are on their way to work (or have limited mobility time), they need to regulate their own time. In addition, some clients, especially those who are vulnerable, may need to learn to be wary of strangers who flatter them to draw them into revealing their names and addresses.

Sometimes the public stops the client to make sure he or she is safe. Learning to educate the public about deaf-blindness can be an important part of O&M, so if the client wants to reassure the other person, he or she should be encouraged to do so. But clients should also learn that they are not obliged to do what the public says or to prolong endless communication and assurances with pedestrians who doubt their ability. Before beginning training in business areas, the instructor should discuss assertiveness (see "Assertiveness with the Public" in Chapter 6).

Many problems that arise during lessons can be avoided if the instructor tells the client the following (using the method or language that the client understands best):

1. At the beginning of each lesson, you and I will decide how close I will be during each part of the lesson.
2. If I approach you during the lesson, I will always immediately give you my signal (name-sign). If someone approaches you without that signal, assume that it is not me.
3. I will often pretend that I do not know you, to allow you to interact by yourself. When you prepare to get assistance to cross streets, I will go away, so you can wait alone.
4. If I need to contact you in an emergency or pull you out of danger, I will try to first give the X signal, so you will know we must act quickly (see "X Signal for Emergencies" in Chapter 2).
5. You should do as much independently as possible during a lesson (though using good judgment), so I am able to observe how you perform the task. However, if it is prudent to seek assistance to accomplish the task, do so; knowing how and when to get assistance is part of independent travel.
6. Sometimes when we are together during mobility lessons, people may approach us to talk to you or me. We need to determine whether you want me to interpret in these situations and if so, how it should be done. One successful strategy is for me to look at you and ask (while interpreting), "A [man, woman, or salesman] is approaching us. Shall I interpret?" Voicing this statement for the other person to hear usually helps the person to understand the situation (see "Interpreting for the Public" in Chapter 3 for the rationale behind this suggestion.)

   If you answer that you want me to interpret, you take the lead; I will be interpreting. You should conclude the conversation yourself, by saying good-bye or that you need to continue your travels or lesson or whatever.
7. When I am interpreting and people are puzzled about why I am not talking with them or they do not understand what I am doing, you should explain my role as interpreter to them (I will interpret your explanation for them). (For the rationale behind this statement, see "Establishing Roles" in Chapter 1.)
8. When interacting with strangers during a lesson, you can take the opportunity to educate the public, but consider the length of the lesson and the time when deciding whether to do so.

An Incident that Could Have Been Avoided

The following story demonstrates the need to establish clear roles for the instructor and client ahead of time and to help the client develop assertiveness and self-confidence.

> One night, I was conducting a lesson with a young college student who had Usher's syndrome. She veered into the street and I followed. After she failed to recognize the situation, I tactilely signed into her hand that she was in the street. When we stepped back onto the curb, a few people gathered, and one man lectured us sternly

about the danger of going into the street (all of which I interpreted tactilely). In response to their questions, my client signed (while I voice interpreted) that I was the instructor, she was learning, and that we were fine. When the man finished his lecture, he turned to the others, introduced himself as a minister, and thanked them.

After they left, I demonstrated to my client how she had veered into the street. We walked into the street, so I could show her how she could recognize the danger next time. The people ran back to us after calling the police. Again, I interpreted everything, answering questions if they were directed to me. "What were you doing in the street?" they demanded, and "Why did you go where we told you not to go?" I explained (while interpreting) that I was showing my client how to avoid that situation. They wanted verification that I was an instructor, which I was unable to produce (even if I had been willing). At one point the minister told me to stop interpreting because it was not to the client, but to me that he wanted to speak (I continued to interpret).

After about 20 minutes of their interrogation and confrontation, I finally asked my client if she was ready to proceed on our trip. She nodded yes. The people then tried to convince her (using me as the interpreter, ironically) to stay until the police arrived. She considered staying, but finally made her way through the throng and we continued with the lesson, followed for a short distance by some of the people. The minister muttered as he finally left, "I guess there's nothing we can do about them." The police never showed up.

This incident occurred before either the client or I was prepared to handle such a situation, and it was thus needlessly prolonged and tense. Because we had not established our roles ahead of time, the client expected that I, as the instructor, would assume control of the situation, but I expected her to take control, since I was interpreting. When I stepped out of my role of interpreter to answer their questions and get involved in the conversation, my role became more unclear to both the client and the other people.

In addition, the client was not confident, and we had not discussed assertiveness or her rights. She seemed to think that these people knew what was best for her. An assertive, confident traveler would perhaps have tried briefly to educate these people about her competence, then would have moved on if they continued to try to stop and protect her (see Chapter 6).

Being Identified as Deaf-Blind

Although it is important that people with whom the deaf-blind person wants to communicate realize that he or she is deaf-blind, it is helpful for others to know as well. Whether or not to identify oneself as deaf-blind to passersby is an individual decision that will be affected by the person's perception of the safety of the surrounding area. Except in dangerous communities, it is sometimes an advantage that others know, because otherwise the deaf-blind traveler suffers the consequences when others assume that he or she understands their verbal warnings. I once interceded when a client was about to hit his head on a conveyer belt that had been set up across the sidewalk to unload a truck; the driver, with his arms full, assumed that the client heard his warnings. Another client was taken to jail for failing to heed the verbal commands of security guards at the airport (see "When the Instructor Should Step In" earlier in this chapter for the complete story). Also, people who try to interact with a deaf-blind person as he or she passes sometimes become irritated when they receive no response and, if the deaf-blind person becomes aware of it, he or she is left puzzled about their angry behavior.

To inform others of their disabilities, people who are deaf-blind can wear a button that says, "I AM DEAF AND BLIND," "I AM DEAF AND VISUALLY IMPAIRED," or "I AM BLIND AND HEARING IMPAIRED." These buttons are available from the Helen Keller National Center for Deaf-Blind Youths and Adults (see "Buttons for Identification" in Resources). Other forms of identification are professionally printed cards inserted in name tag holders stating that the wearers are deaf-blind and explaining how to communicate. Occasionally, these strategies are effective, but usually the public either does not understand them or realizes what they mean only after they have left the person who is deaf-blind.

Naturally, it is the deaf-blind person's decision whether to try to let others know that he or she is deaf-blind and if so, in what manner. The instructor's role is to inform the client how his or her presence and behavior affects others, including whether people become perplexed or angry when the client does not respond to them. People who decide to try to inform the public about their deafness can work with the instructor to find out the most effective ways for them.

If the person's speech is understandable, others often fail to realize that he or she is deaf. During our recent surveys of people who helped a deaf-blind person cross the street, most people recognized that the person was deaf when he used sign language while speaking (Sauerburger & Jones, 1992). It would be interesting to see if this strategy is effective for other people who are deaf-blind.

CHAPTER 5

ISOLATION

One Wednesday evening on my way home from orienting Chris Cook, a deaf-blind student, to the campus of Gallaudet University, I heard over the radio that Operation Desert Storm had begun and our country was at war. I worked with Chris again Friday and the following Monday. Since Monday was a holiday, I asked if he had been able to keep up with the news of the war that day.

"What war?" he asked.

The insulation of deaf-blind people from the outside world can be considerable, even for busy college students who are on campus where most people know how to communicate with them. Why is this the case?

FACTORS CONTRIBUTING TO ISOLATION

Some methods of communicating with people who are deaf-blind must be done individually and are more tedious than other people are accustomed to. Tactile communication can also involve touching and intimacy that make some people uncomfortable. Thus, even people who know how to communicate often do not bother to discuss with the deaf-blind person what they would have discussed if communication were easier. Other people, including some family members and former friends, do not know how to do so.

For example, I have observed that often family members—parents, spouses, and even children—of deaf people whose primary language is sign language cannot sign. This problem is common (Duncan et al., 1988). Thus, communication with families often is limited even for deaf people who can see. If the person cannot see or loses vision, many family members are not able or willing to learn new methods to communicate with him or her.

THIS CHAPTER WAS WRITTEN IN COLLABORATION WITH PSYCHOLOGISTS MCCAY VERNON, PH.D., JEAN BAYARD, PH.D., AND ROBERT BAYARD, PH.D.

This problem was repeatedly raised by deaf-blind people who were interviewed by Yoken (1979). The situation of Joan, who had impaired hearing and vision, was typical and is described in the following observations:

> Even with her parents, who are otherwise extremely supportive of her and with whom she enjoys a good relationship, communication becomes a frustration. She has tried to get them to learn sign language . . . ; she has urged them, both verbally and with illustrated cards taped to the refrigerator, to learn fingerspelling . . . . In what probably describes many family relationships for hearing impaired individuals, she says, "They understand how serious the problem is, but they don't understand how serious the problem is, if you know what I mean." When she misses a large part of the dinner table conversation, Joan and her mother will sit down together later and "rehash" what was said. Joan seems to reconcile herself to the situation partly with the feeling that much of what she misses is either repetitive or not particularly interesting (Yoken, p. 74).

It is surprising that many deaf people and blind people are also reluctant to interact with people who are deaf-blind. It would seem that being either deaf or blind would help prepare a person to understand or feel comfortable in the presence of people who have both a visual and a hearing impairment. Yet when the person who is deaf or who is blind becomes deaf-blind, he or she is often ignored or misunderstood by fellow deaf people or blind people. Also, as mobility instructor Barbara Seever pointed out, professionals in the fields of deafness and blindness (some of whom are blind or deaf themselves) are afraid to work with deaf-blind people.

The most common explanation of why people who are deaf or blind avoid deaf-blind people is that they are terrified of becoming deaf-blind themselves. From what I have observed, however, the more likely reason is that they are just as perplexed and reluctant as anyone else to get involved with people who have other disabilities, especially when the disability makes communication difficult. For example, one person who is deaf and losing her vision told me, "I noticed some deaf people as well as 'hearies' don't feel like doing anything special to communicate with deaf-blind people, like tactile signs. Some are uncomfortable doing this. Other deaf people have no patience to sign more slowly than their natural speed." After her interviews, Yoken (1979, p. 27) speculated that "the deaf-blind person's loss of contact [with other deaf people], though nonetheless painful, may also be a drifting away; the deaf community's reaction, [may be] a forgetting rather than an abrupt and callous rejection."

However, it is not just family members, friends, and other disabled people who have difficulty overcoming their reluctance to interact with the person who is deaf-blind. It is also difficult for neighbors, classmates and teachers, agency staff, potential employers, and the public to be willing to do so because they do not know how or do not want to learn how to communicate. People who are deaf-blind often find themselves at a job or residential setting or school where they are left alone because few or no people are able or willing to interact with them. One man who became deaf and blind as an adult told Yoken (p.53): "I learned to discard a lot of people with my deafness. The situation now is that people who want to communicate with me have to put out some effort themselves. I can't do it all myself. And it can be damned hard work to communicate with me. I've had to find out who the people are who are willing to crank out all the energy it takes, and do it over time . . . ."

The accumulated effect of this restriction of information can be formidable and, as Yoken (pp. 157–158) said, "can redirect an individual's experiences in unfathomable ways. Isolation is an unavoidable reality in the lives of deaf-blind people. For most, the loneliness and alienation is massive and unrelieved. One theme emerging from the interviews is the relationship among rejection, withdrawal, and isolation. One way that people deal with rejection, obvious or subtle, is to avoid the contact that makes it possible. . . . The longer any individual remains detached from a group, the more difficult it becomes for the group to include him, and the more painful it becomes for him to risk further rejection."

The rejection felt by people who are deaf-blind may or may not be intentional. With limited awareness of what other people are doing or feeling, it is easy to misconstrue a lack of interaction or a miscommunication. Yoken (p. 159) said that with insufficient feedback from others about their feelings, "the deaf-blind person loses an accurate perception of the validity of multiple points of view and of what are reasonable expectations of others."

The capacity of people to tolerate isolation is far in excess of what could be imagined. As psychologist Vernon McCay, cited in Duncan et al. (1988, p. 58) noted, however, it is vitally important to maintain communication with the person who is deaf-blind in order to avoid his or her "withdrawal, increased egocentricity, and breakdown in the remaining human relationships."

REDUCING ISOLATION

Educating Others

It is important, then, to help those who may come in contact regularly with the deaf-blind person to be comfortable interacting with him or her. Family members, friends, co-workers, and caretakers can be encouraged to make the adjustment to new methods of communication and be given opportunities to learn them.

In-service training or special classes can help people learn how to interact with the person who is deaf-blind. If possible, deaf-blind people should organize their own in-service or training so that others will learn about their particular needs, and so that they will become experienced advocating for themselves and teaching others how to interact comfortably with them.

When a person's visual field is reduced, as it is with Usher's syndrome, it can be difficult for others to understand how to interact. In working with adolescents with

Usher's syndrome, Vernon and Hicks (1983) learned that the adolescents' peers seemed to understand and be supportive of their problems with night blindness, but not with tunnel vision. When their friends waved or signed to the visually impaired students and the students did not respond, they thought the students were intentionally ignoring them or being "stupid." Yoken's (1979, p. 82) interviewees reported the same thing; one said that in school, a lot of the children "didn't understand. Sometimes they're waving at me and they think I'm ignoring them or acting ugly."

I found, however, that even service providers do not always understand the implications of tunnel vision. One teacher in a day program for adults who are deaf and mentally retarded said that before receiving in-service training, she had thought her student was faking blindness. Since the teacher knew only that the student was supposed to be "visually impaired" with "tunnel vision," she had signed close to her face, but the student seemed to not understand her. Yet the teacher observed that the student could easily see and understand signs from friends across the room.

Often, the most effective way to explain the effects of a reduced visual field is for people to try low vision simulators that resemble the particular deaf-blind person's vision. After using simulators, this teacher finally understood why her student could not understand when she signed close to her and experimented to find how she could communicate better. The low vision simulators can be made inexpensively. For example, the screw-in lens of welding goggles can be replaced with cardboard with an appropriate-sized hole to simulate reduced visual field. One eye must be occluded while the other looks through the simulator. To simulate the loss of central vision or visual acuity, the goggle lens can be smeared appropriately with fingernail polish (Sauerburger, 1991).

Enhancing the Environment

Some people are isolated because they live or spend every day with family members or institutional staff who seem unable or unwilling to overcome the communication barrier. The family or staff may be reluctant to make the effort, but they need to realize that the person may suffer severe isolation if they do not. If the situation does not improve, it may be best for the deaf-blind person to move to an environment (or at least spend time regularly) where people are comfortable interacting and communicating with him or her and where the isolation can be decreased.

Many people who are deaf-blind have found that they can decrease their isolation and dependence by moving to a metropolitan area. Cities offer more accessible public transportation, community activities, and services that can include deaf-blind people and meet their needs. Places with large communities of other deaf and deaf-blind people offer more opportunities to interact with those who share their culture and language. Seattle has a large population of people who are deaf-blind and offers many services, such as interpreting and public transportation.

At the 1992 Hilton-Perkins Deaf-Blind Conference, presenters who are deaf-blind explained how they improved their lives and decreased their isolation by moving to Seattle. When they lived in their hometowns with their families, they were unable to get anywhere without the assistance of others who could drive. Interaction with friends, co-workers, and even family members was limited because of the communication barrier, and job opportunities were poor. After moving to Seattle, they were able to live independently and travel using public transportation, were accepted as part of the community, and had extensive contact with people who share their language and culture.

Deaf-blind people who live in residential institutions or attend day programs are often grouped with people who are blind or who have disabilities other than deafness. However, they would benefit most from being with those who can communicate with them. For many deaf-blind people who primarily use signs or gestures, this means being with other deaf people and staff who are familiar with this communication. If they are grouped with people who have other disabilities, their interaction with staff and peers is usually limited.

Usually the goal of rehabilitation is for the person to live independently. For many people this means living by themselves. I have spoken with people who are blind or deaf-blind who struggled to become independent, only to live alone for many years, becoming more and more isolated. One deaf-blind man had lived in an apartment for 15 years and did not know who his neighbors were. Others have told me how lonely they became after achieving their independence. Many nevertheless prefer to live alone, but efforts need to be made for them to be included in activities and to have contact with others.

Deaf-blind clubs that have been organized throughout the country have numerous advantages, not only for deaf-blind people, but for their families and friends. These clubs should be organized and run by deaf-blind people and not by service providers, whose role should be to facilitate the contacts needed to get the group started, provide information and support services (such as interpreting), and refer people to the groups. The club in metropolitan Washington, DC, which meets one evening a month, sometimes has speakers and sometimes has recreational or other activities. In addition, it hosts an annual picnic and campouts and publishes a quarterly newsletter. Interpretive and support services are provided by friends (many of whom are deaf), family members, and interested service providers. The majority of the board members and the president have both visual and hearing impairments. For information on and assistance in starting a group, contact the American Association of the Deaf-Blind (see Resources).

Increasing Communication

To lessen the information gap that can occur because of limited communication, the worker should do everything possible to allow the person who is deaf-blind to experience the world around him or her. Point out or describe the environment as fully as possible, including signs of current events, new trends, and fashions, and share news about major events. For example, mobility instructor Barbara Seever was about to begin a lesson with a deaf-blind woman when the space shuttle Challenger blew up. When Barbara asked, her client told her that she knew about the launch, and they spent the next hour listening for more news from the radio while Barbara interpreted. After they proceeded with the lesson, they stopped many times to talk as Barbara heard more news come in.

A common complaint of deaf-blind people is that others do not greet them or inform them that they are present. They find out later that a friend or acquaintance was in the same room or passed without talking to them. During a speech at Radcliffe College, where she was studying for a bachelor's degree, Helen Keller said (quoted in Lash, 1980, p. 275), "I have had moments of loneliness when the girls have passed me on the stairs and in the lecture-rooms without a sign. I have sometimes had a depressing sense of isolation in the midst of my classmates. There are times when one wearies of books, which after all are only symbols of the spirit, and when one reaches out to the warm, living touch of a friendly hand. But I understand perfectly how the girls feel. They cannot speak to me, and they do not see the light of recognition in my face as we pass. The situation to them must be strange and discouraging." Make the effort to let the person who is deaf-blind know that you are near or passing by. If you encounter him or her often, the two of you may make up a signal, such as a special tap on the elbow, that you can use to announce your presence easily.

People who live alone can reduce the isolation by arranging for volunteers to help with such tasks as reading mail, shopping, discussing news events, or providing companionship. Some areas have organizations that recruit and train volunteers, or the deaf-blind person can advertise for assistance.

Increasing the Person's Effectiveness

As beneficial as it may be for the worker to adapt the environment and help others be more comfortable with the person who is deaf-blind, it is even more important for deaf-blind people to know how to advocate for themselves, establish good communication, and put others at ease. For example, it usually falls to the person who is deaf-blind to inform others of his or her needs and desires. When Geraldine Lawhorn, who is deaf-blind, attended a camp for blind people, she described in a letter to a deaf-blind friend her efforts to reduce what she calls "that 'Deaf-Blind Isolation.'" She wrote: "Some counselors gave me only important announcements, while those with more insight shared camp news and jokes. When the counselors realized I derived pleasure or benefit from their interpreting, they included me more. One question often asked is, 'What can a deaf-blind person get out of it?' We must respond and show our friends that we get a great deal out of life with the right kind of assistance" (Lawhorn, 1991, p. 137).

Sometimes when the person who is deaf-blind has difficulty establishing communication with others, the problem is that he or she assumes that people already know how to adjust their communication for him or her, but for some reason are not doing it. The deaf-blind person may lament the insensitivity or lack of consideration of people whose signs are too large or too close for his or her reduced visual field or who exaggerate their lip movement in vain attempts to be understood. One visually impaired woman was reluctant to let others know that it was painful when they spoke loudly into her hearing aid. She was depressed because of the isolation her loss of hearing was causing, but she preferred to avoid interacting with people who unknowingly inflicted the pain on her, rather than explain to them how to communicate with her comfortably. People who are deaf-blind need to realize that others have to be told exactly what to do, often repeatedly.

Another problem is that some deaf-blind people do not know that others need to use a different approach to communicate with them. Some people whose experience is limited to familiar people do not realize that those people are using communication techniques that are unknown to the public. Others are unaware of how their vision and hearing differs from that of other people. For example, in working with adolescents with Usher's syndrome, Vernon and Hicks (1983) found that the students had difficulties because when they did not see their friends' greetings, the friends thought they were being intentionally ignored. Rather than conduct an in-service session to explain it to the entire school, Vernon and Hicks chose to educate the students about their own vision. "For the first time in their lives, [the students] understood in practical terms how their vision differed from the vision of others. Thus they were able to describe the problem to friends and explain how to get their attention." (Vernon & Hicks, p. 65). Just as teaching a hungry man how to fish can feed him for a lifetime, helping people who are deaf-blind learn how to advocate for themselves can be much more effective than trying to do it for them.

Adjusting to Isolation

Some deaf-blind people despair that they will always be alone and lonely. One young deaf woman thought that no man would ever be interested in dating or marrying her if he knew she was becoming blind. The perception that no one would marry a person who is deaf-blind is strong. Yet I know dozens of deaf-blind men and women who are married, many of whom met their spouses after they became deaf-blind. They are happily involved with their families, do their share of household chores, and in some cases raise children.

When I met the young woman again several years later, she was happily married. I asked her what I should tell other deaf-blind people when they are in the depths of despair as she was. She said to tell them about her experience and to assure them that she learned that people can be accepted and loved by others as unique human beings, regardless of whether they have vision and hearing.

It may help people who are rejected by others to know that usually the rejection is not personal, but a result of the others' fear or ignorance of deaf-blindness. They need to realize that interaction with others frequently requires considerable patience and understanding. Sometimes they are so caught up in the rejection and awkwardness of the situation that they are unaware of the great patience, courage, and personal strength that they had developed to deal with it. Recognition of their efforts and abilities can be encouraging to them as they try to overcome the barriers of dealing with others.

During her interviews, Yoken (1979) learned that for some people, religious faith was the primary source of support for adjusting to their deaf-blindness. Also, in religious communities, such as churches or synagogues, many isolated people found others who were willing to accept and communicate with them.

People often find it easier to handle the increased isolation, frustration, and hurt that can result from trying to interact with others if they talk with other people who are deaf-blind, especially well-adjusted role models. Knowing that they are not alone in their struggles and that people who are deaf-blind can lead happy, productive lives can be extremely helpful. If you cannot find such people in the community, contact the American Association of the Deaf-Blind, an active consumer organization established by deaf-blind people (see "Consumer Organizations" in Resources). The association has several local clubs across the country; holds an annual convention that is usually an uplifting experience for both deaf-blind persons and for those who attend as helpers; and publishes a quarterly magazine, *The Deaf-Blind American,* that includes articles by and for people who are deaf-blind.

HALLUCINATIONS: A CONSEQUENCE OF SEVERE ISOLATION

While working or becoming acquainted with over 75 people who are deaf-blind, I knew seven who hallucinated or had hallucinated in the past. At first, I mistakenly thought that their hallucinations were a sign of psychiatric or neurological problems.

Of these seven people, two had other symptoms of psychiatric problems for which they were receiving counseling and that probably were the cause of their hallucinations. A third person had Alzheimer's disease. These people were not profoundly deaf and totally blind; they could still understand speech under good conditions, and two had good functional vision. The remaining four had no other symptoms of psychiatric disorders. They all were lucid and showed no signs of dementia. However, they were profoundly deaf, had limited vision, and led isolated lives. The physical movement of two of them was limited by confinement to a wheelchair. Their hallucinations were most likely caused by isolation and sensory deprivation.

Two of these people were women who lived in nursing homes, and two were men. One of the women asked me to help her arrange to visit the farm that she said her doctor had bequeathed to her. It took me several weeks, during which I tried to locate the farm, before I realized it was imaginary. Later, she confided to me that she was eloping soon with a secret lover who visited her frequently, and eventually during our sessions she began talking with people who were not there. The other woman also chatted frequently with people who were not there. The older man who lived in a group home had an exciting imaginary life as a member of a secret police organization and often told stories about his adventures (whether or not anyone was there to listen). The second man, who was born profoundly deaf and had lost all but a little central vision as an adult, had regularly experienced frightening hallucinations of monsters in the past.

Why Some People Hallucinate

The sensory input of people who are profoundly deaf and totally or nearly totally blind is severely constricted, and the lives of some of them are extremely isolated. According to Slade and Bentall (1988), hallucinations are common among people who are isolated for long periods, especially under stress. Mountain climbers, arctic explorers, and lone sailors and pilots have reported having hallucinations. Hostages have reported having had visual imagery experiences, including some complex memory images, and two miners who were trapped in darkness for two days reported seeing visions of such things as doorways and stairs and even the pope.

Many normal persons experience hallucinations while they are drifting off to sleep. In the 1950s, researchers discovered to their surprise that of the people they studied who were cut off from sensory stimulation for just a few hours, over half saw images and some eventually hallucinated integrated scenes (Mendelson et al., 1964; Slade & Bentall, 1988; Solomon et al., 1965; Zubek, 1969). Furthermore, the effects of sensory deprivation are increased by restricted movement (see Appendix B for further information).

Thus the hallucinations of people who are deaf-blind are not necessarily a sign of psychosis. Instead, they could be a symptom of isolation and sensory deprivation, perhaps intensified by limited physical movement.

Of the four people who had no other symptoms of psychiatric problems but who hallucinated, three were totally blind or nearly so. After they lost their hearing, they were not able to communicate effectively with anyone regularly for months or years. Our agency provided training in communication methods, both for the deaf-blind people and for the staff at the facilities where they lived. However, the three continue to hallucinate and seem to enjoy their imaginary lives as much as or more than their real lives.

The service provider who worked with the man who had the frightening hallucinations did not focus on the hallucinations, but rather encouraged him to become more involved and experience life. The man eventually got a job and an apartment and found friends, some of whom were deaf or deaf-blind, who were able to communicate easily with him. The hallucinations diminished until, by the time I met him, he no longer was troubled by them.

What Should the Worker Do?

People who normally have no symptoms of psychiatric or neurological problems but who hallucinate while undergoing experimental sensory deprivation or while stranded or isolated under stress are not referred for psychiatric therapy. Rather, their hallucinations end when the sensory deprivation or isolation ends. Likewise, if the deaf-blind person has no symptoms of psychiatric problems other than harmless hallucinations or delusions, there is probably no need to refer him or her for counseling or psychiatric therapy. If the hallucinations are caused by isolation and sensory deprivation, they can be reduced by reducing the isolation and sensory deprivation. Referral for diagnosis and possible treatment would be appropriate if the person has psychological problems or symptoms of neurological disorders in addition to the hallucinations or if the hallucinations are disturbing to the person. If the hallucinations are the result of psychosis, they are best managed by psychiatric treatment, including antihallucinogenic medication.

If the person considers the hallucinations to be a problem, he or she can reduce their occurrence by becoming involved in enjoyable activities, especially those that are mentally challenging. Attempts should be made to improve the quality and quantity of communication between the deaf-blind person and other people and to help the person establish companionship. When the person begins to engage in sufficient activities and meaningful contact with others, the imaginary experiences may diminish. In the meantime, the person may resist giving up the imaginary world without having worthwhile alternatives in the real world. It may be helpful for him or her to realize that this phenomenon is shared by others, both deaf-blind and hearing sighted, who experience sensory deprivation or isolation.

In cases in which people have delusions, such as that of the client who imagined he was a member of a secret police organization, a standard treatment is to help the client encapsulate what is imaginary, that is, to retain the delusional system but not let it interfere with other aspects of life. Many people function successfully in life with well-encapsulated delusional and hallucinatory systems.

If the deaf-blind person enjoys the hallucinations or delusions, the worker should accept them. We all confront difficulties with a variety of coping mechanisms, some of which are healthy and some of which are counterproductive. Having hallucinations is one way of coping with isolation. In some respects, it is a healthy alternative to suffering from sensory deprivation and isolation. People in many non-Western cultures consider hallucinations a positive experience and for centuries have induced them through hypnosis, drugs, isolation, and fasting as a way of getting in touch with their inner or spiritual selves (Hultkrantz, 1987; Slade & Bentall, 1988).

If the person tries to involve you in the imaginary world or asks questions about it, you can explain that although he or she may be aware of the people, things, or animals, you and others cannot see or hear them. You should not pretend that the imaginary world exists anywhere but in the person's mind, but it also does little good to try to make him or her realize that it is not real or to deny the existence of the hallucinations. To that person, they may be real. If the hallucinations are interfering with the person's concentration on a lesson or task, ask him or her either to ignore them for the time being or to request the people or animals to leave for now.

CHAPTER 6

ASSERTIVENESS AND CONTROL OVER ONE'S LIFE

True independence usually requires assertiveness and the ability to make decisions. Yet many people who are deaf-blind have limited opportunities to develop assertiveness and decision-making skills. Decisions are often made for them, and they are not given access to the information they would need to make those decisions.

Sometimes access to information is intentionally cut off. Peggy Lamb (Lamb, 1989, p. 26), who is deaf-blind, explained what happened to her:

> I would like to share with you a few incidents to show you some of the obstacles I have had to overcome because I am deaf and blind—starting with my husband's death. The welfare department would not help him because he was Catholic. The Catholic people did help, but they did not tell me what the doctors told them! I was led up the garden path. I was not told he had cancer! When the hospital wanted to move him to a hospice, the doctor sent for me to explain, but the priest interpreting did not tell me what they said. [Later] I wrote the hospital and asked why I had not been told everything. The doctor and hospital staff were angry for me and complained about it to those helping and supporting me. So the people who had helped me threatened me and said they would do no more.

Any person who is experienced in working with people who are deaf-blind can probably tell similar stories. For example, the family of one of my clients refused to tell him that his brother, to whom he was close, was dying. When his brother finally died, a staff worker had to inform him.

These are extreme examples of what regularly happens to people who are deaf-blind. Unpleasant truths are withheld, presumably to protect the person, on the assumption that he or she is not as capable of coping with the truth as are other people. At other times, the information is not provided to the person because it is too time consuming or difficult to do so.

As a result, decisions are often made for people who are deaf-blind, sometimes without so much as consulting or informing them. As Boyd Wolfe, who is deaf-blind, said, "Too many times, people are inclined to try to make up our minds for us. They think that they know what's best for us and we know nothing. This is even done in some cases by the 'professionals' who work with us, though this conduct is not at all professional."

Disabled or not, most people have some problems with others' trying to make their decisions or take over for them. However, the difficulties are compounded for persons who are deaf-blind because of their double sensory impairment and their dependence on others to get the information needed to make their own decisions.

For example, one deaf man who lost his vision noticed that the communication barrier made people less willing to ask him about decisions. In a typical incident, his sister was guiding him through a hotel but then stopped and asked him to wait for a moment. Since he knew the layout of the hotel, he correctly guessed that she was hesitant about his using the escalator and was looking for the elevator. He later explained, "I know if I was hearing, she would have simply asked and talked about this with me. Although she knew fingerspelling and was using it effectively with me, she was feeling hesitant to ask me and went on. . .to make her own decision. I quickly caught on and asked her if she was concerned about my going on the escalator." This man strongly believes that the deaf-blind person needs to be more assertive than the hearing-blind or the sighted-deaf person.

The effect of the sensory deprivation itself may also contribute to a deaf-blind person's lack of assertiveness, although the results of experiments with people undergoing temporary sensory deprivation may not be applicable to deaf-blind people who have adjusted to the disability. Studies show that some people who undergo experimental deprivation of both vision and hearing become more susceptible to the experimenter's suggestions and persuasion because of their strong desire for information and sensory stimulation (see Appendix B).

CONSEQUENCES OF LOSS OF CONTROL

Some people who are deaf-blind become accustomed to having information withheld and decisions made for them, although, according to psychologist McCay Vernon, people in this situation may experience hostile dependence and other psychological and emotional consequences. Other deaf-blind persons are wary of people's tendencies to make decisions for them. As Lawhorn (1991, p. 131), who is deaf-blind, wrote, "How could I make people understand the difference between helping and 'taking over'? The take-over type says, 'I fixed the picture on your wall; it was upside down.' The helper says, 'The picture on your wall is upside down. Shall I adjust it—or do you prefer to display your photos upside down like certain magazines do?' Laughing with the helper, *I* can make the decision." Patrick Murphy, a consultant on deaf-blindness for Britain's National Deaf-Blind League and himself deaf-blind, stated at the league's 1989 convention, "It can be only too easy for a guide-helper of the wrong temperament to dominate a deaf-blind person" (Murphy, 1989).

This happened even to Helen Keller. When she was young, her family thwarted her plans to marry because they thought that the marriage would not be wise. Even when she was a competent woman in her 40s, her companion, Anne Sullivan Macy, withheld a letter from an admirer who proposed marriage until she could investigate and approve of the suitor (Lash, 1980). Warren Bledsoe, one of the originators of O&M, told me of another such incident in Helen Keller's life (personal correspondence, 1991). Miss Keller wanted to go to the airport to greet Henry Wallace, who was vice president of the United States and a controversial figure. Those around her told Bledsoe that she might be photographed by the *New York Times* while greeting Wallace with a hug and a kiss and that it would be politically unwise for her, so they procrastinated until she had to abandon her plans to meet Wallace then.

Many people who are deaf-blind have had similar experiences when decisions are made by those who "know what is best" for them or who find it too tiresome to inform them of the choices that are available. These decisions may be simple, such as what to choose from a menu, or major, such as whom to marry or whether to marry.

I sometimes forget about the tendency of others to make decisions for deaf-blind people. For example, a woman who was arranging for speakers for the annual convention of her professional organization called to ask me to help her find a volunteer to stay at the hotel with a presenter who was deaf-blind. The presenter apparently was capable, and the caller had already arranged transportation from the airport to the hotel, as well as an interpreter for the convention. When I asked why the deaf-blind woman would need additional round-the-clock companionship, I was told that she had requested it. Still puzzled, I suggested that she be asked what the volunteer's role would be. The woman agreed to call her again.

Later the mystery was solved when I learned that the woman had never communicated directly with the presenter, but rather with her colleague, who explained that it was she who had requested the volunteer, not the presenter herself. The colleague admitted that the deaf-blind woman had tried (apparently in vain) to reassure her that she had traveled alone many times and that she would be fine by herself.

I should have been alert to the possibility that the woman who called me had never spoken directly with the deaf-blind woman and that the deaf-blind woman had not been consulted about getting a volunteer companion. Like most people who make decisions for deaf-blind people, the colleague thought she was well intentioned ("It is the mother instinct in me," she explained), when she was actually being patronizing. But the result was the same—the deaf-blind woman's potential loss of control over her life and decisions.

Situations like these can be avoided when people make it a point to find out how they can communicate directly with the deaf-blind person (such as through TDD, the mail, or an interpreter). If direct communication is not possible, they should ask that the person who is deaf-blind be informed of the communication and consulted, rather than let someone else speak for him or her.

GAINING CONTROL OVER ONE'S LIFE

People who are deaf-blind can take more control over their lives by

- recognizing their ability and their right to make their own decisions;
- developing good communication skills for use with the public and strangers, as well as with familiar people;
- establishing dependable sources of the information on which they need to base their decisions (including friends, volunteers, agencies, interpreters, technology, and accessible media);
- learning safe, effective techniques for independent living and traveling;
- practicing making decisions and solving problems;
- improving self-confidence with successful experiences;
- becoming skilled at helping others to understand more about people who are deaf-blind and to be comfortable interacting with them (individually, as with potential employers, or in groups, such as providing sensitivity training and workshops about deaf-blindness); and
- learning to advocate for themselves and their needs.

Applying these behaviors and principles is not always easy, and help from a service provider can sometimes be instrumental. For example, one problem that Vernon and Hicks (1983) discussed in group sessions with students who had Usher's syndrome at the Model Secondary School for the Deaf in Washington, DC, was that the students could not see well while waiting with their classmates in the dim halls at mealtimes; they bumped into others and had to ask them to repeat their signs. The students had resigned themselves to the inevitability of these difficulties. To their surprise, the problems were eliminated simply by having the lighting improved in the halls and dormitories. Seeing the positive results of constructive action gave them a sense of control over their lives.

Some deaf-blind people think they would like to get a new job, move away from parents or out of an institution, or get involved in community activities, but they have no idea how to get started, what is available, or even what such a decision might entail. People around them give advice about what they think would be best, but often the deaf-blind persons do not have access to information on which to make their own decisions. This situation can be frustrating and increase their feelings of isolation, helplessness, and loss of contact with reality. People whose vision and hearing are severely limited usually need someone dependable, such as a friend, family member, volunteer, or service provider, to help them get the information without trying to influence their decisions.

The role of the service provider is to encourage people to make their own decisions. For example, the deaf-blind person who wants to live on his or her own can be shown what it would mean (such as cooking and shopping for oneself). Rather than abstract discussions of the skills needed, the deaf-blind person may need opportunities to use these skills. He or she can then realize what skills are needed for such a move and decide whether it is worth learning them. If the person thinks that the goal is achievable, the service provider could help him or her arrange for transportation and an interpreter to read real estate ads, talk to a real estate agent, compare costs with income, look at available apartments or homes and see if the neighborhood has available shopping and commuting opportunities.

Sometimes it is easy to dismiss the deaf-blind person's desires as unrealistic and to encourage him or her to do what you "know" is best. However, the decision must be that person's. Your role is to provide all the information needed; you need to overcome any temptation to manage the deaf-blind person and make decisions for him or her. If the deaf-blind person has the information about what such a choice would involve and what other choices are available, he or she may agree that the aspiration is unrealistic. Conversely, he or she may make a bad decision. We all have the right to make our own mistakes. It is the best way to learn about life, and it helps us make better decisions in the future. Even if the deaf-blind person makes a decision of which the helper does not approve, that may be the decision with which the deaf-blind person is happy.

ASSERTIVENESS WITH THE PUBLIC

Independent travelers who are deaf-blind often find it difficult to be assertive with the well-meaning but uninformed public. People will try to guide them where they think they want to go or may call the police to protect them. The ability to communicate with the public should be developed as much as possible, since its absence is often what impels the public to take action on behalf of the deaf-blind person. In addition, before the client begins mobility training in business areas, I discuss assertiveness and offer the following suggestions (using the method or language he or she understands best):

1. Only you know what is best for you. Do not assume that others understand and know what is best for you.
2. You know when you need help and what kind of help is best.
3. If people offer you help that you are not sure you need, you can use the method or methods of communication that you use with the public to ask for more information (Why do they want to help you? Is there a danger or problem of which you were unaware?). With this information *you* decide if you need their help or not.

4. If people insist on helping when you do not need it:

a. Act confident (even if you are not), and smile reassuringly.

b. If this is a recurring problem, prepare a card that explains that you can travel independently.

c. If all else fails, just move away from them and continue on your way. You are *not* obligated to convince them that you do not need assistance, nor are you required to accept their help even if *they* think that you need it.

5. If you choose to be guided, you will assume better control if you take the person's arm, rather than let the person take your arm. Review the Hines break for this purpose (see Glossary).

If the deaf-blind person has poor communication skills and people repeatedly try to intervene, a card can be prepared saying something like, "I can travel independently, but thank you for your concern. You can print letters on my palm with your fingertip." One deaf visually impaired man with nystagmus (quivering eye movement) and staggering gait was repeatedly stopped by the police and brought to the station because people thought he was drunk. He now carries a letter from his physician explaining that this is his normal appearance.

Some people with low self-esteem or with little self-confidence cling to the belief that the public knows what is best for them. When clients and I had discussions after a few incidents in which well-meaning people took them in the wrong direction (often then abandoning them or calling the police because they could not communicate), they usually developed the assertiveness needed to keep the public from taking control. Realizing that the public is usually uninformed can help travelers gain more confidence in their ability to make their own decisions.

CHAPTER 7

ORIENTATION AND MOBILITY TRAINING

This chapter is written for O&M specialists who teach blind and visually impaired people how to travel independently. They may be surprised to realize that except for specialized communication techniques, they probably already know the majority of what they need to teach deaf-blind people to travel independently. Most of the techniques and concerns are the same when teaching deaf-blind and hearing-blind people.

Although it is tempting to generalize about the limits of independence that can be achieved by people who are deaf-blind, each deaf-blind person, like each hearing-blind person, will achieve his or her own level of independence and comfort as a traveler. Some people who are deaf-blind use public transportation or taxis to go anywhere in their city—indeed, anywhere in the country or the world—while others travel alone only on familiar routes or never travel alone. People who are developmentally disabled, deaf, and visually impaired use public transportation to commute independently to their day programs or work. One wheelchair user who is totally blind with a moderate hearing loss commutes to work, takes taxis to new places, and travels around the country by herself. The limits of independence should be imposed not by assumptions of what a person is able to achieve, but by the person's motivation and abilities.

O&M programs for deaf-blind people are similar to those for hearing-blind people. The following major differences are discussed in detail elsewhere in this book:

1. A different method of communication may be used for teaching (see Chapter 1 and Chapter 2 and Figures 1A and B in this chapter).
2. The deaf-blind person may need to develop effective ways of communicating with the public (see Chapter 3).
3. Street-crossing strategies are often different from those of the hearing-blind person (see Chapter 8).

4. The instructor places a greater emphasis on helping the deaf-blind client understand the reaction of the public, by reporting to him or her what happened during the lesson (see "Understanding the Public's Reaction" in Chapter 4).

ADAPTATIONS OF MOBILITY TECHNIQUES

Sighted Guide Technique

I was once amused when another mobility instructor approached me at a convention of the American Association of the Deaf-Blind and said, "I have never *seen* so many awful sighted guide techniques!" These techniques were different from the traditional sighted guide technique, partly because helpers at these conventions have a background in deafness, not in blindness, and thus are not aware of the proper sighted guide techniques and partly because, to facilitate communication while walking, one has to be creative in developing new sighted guide techniques.

In general, any technique with which you and the deaf-blind person are comfortable and that enables him or her to move safely is acceptable. One way to communicate while guiding is to have the deaf-blind person's left hand hold your arm above the elbow in the proper position while his or her right hand is on your right hand to feel the signs. This technique allows the deaf-blind person to feel the movement of your body, so he or she can anticipate drop-offs and turns while communicating. However, it leaves the deaf-blind person with no hands free to hold a cane, purse, or whatever.

If I want to communicate while guiding, I usually have the deaf-blind person's left hand on my right hand to feel my signs as we walk (I sign with my right hand). This technique is also effective when people are exploring a new area because they can follow the wall or rail or explore landmarks with their right hand or cane while I commu-

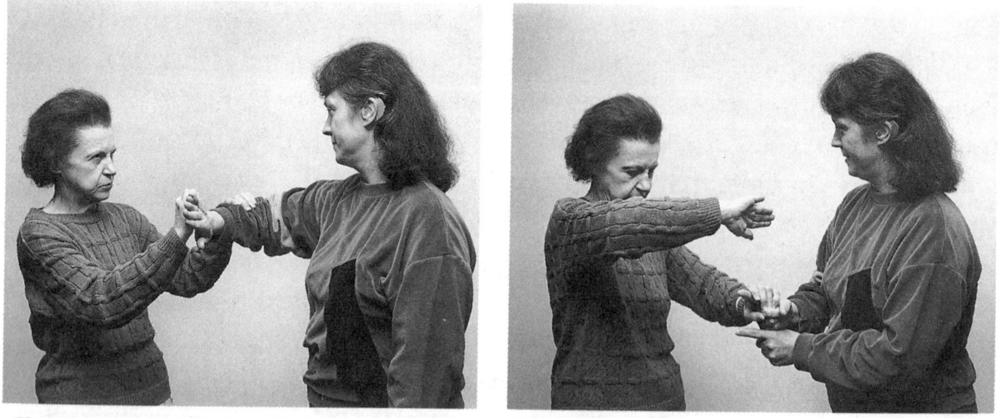

Figures 1A and B. People who cannot see a technique being demonstrated are usually able to follow the demonstration by touch. In 1A here, the deaf-blind woman on the left learns the position of the upper hand and forearm technique by tactilely observing the instructor's demonstration. In 1B, the instructor signs "Correct!" into the woman's left hand as the woman tries the technique herself.

nicate information into their left hand. (If the person is left-handed and you can sign with your left hand, it may be easier to switch sides.)

Guiding in this manner, however, does not give the deaf-blind person adequate warning of stairs, partly because the deaf-blind person is walking by my side and partly because the person cannot feel the movement of my body (my hand does not necessarily go up or down when my body does). One solution is to communicate that stairs are ahead, but then the person does not know how far ahead. Another solution is to stop signing and place the person's hand back on my arm in the proper position above the elbow.

If we are approaching a single step (such as a curb), however, I usually do not bother to switch arm positions, but allow the person to feel my movement and walk a little behind while his or her hand is still on mine. To do so, when we approach the curb, I stop signing, slow down, and bend my elbow back to bring my hand to my side (with the person's hand still on mine). This gesture causes the person to walk a little behind me (in the same position as with the normal sighted guide technique). If I keep my arm rigid when I turn or step up or down, my hand turns or moves up or down with my body, so the person can feel me step up or down and can tell how far ahead the step is.

Mobility instructor Mary Michaud-Cooney pointed out that there are times when the guide's attention should be on where he or she is going, not on communication. When your full concentration is needed, inform the deaf-blind person that the communication needs to be suspended while you negotiate the street or stairs or a tricky congested area. When you can relax again, indicate that you can resume communication.

Cane Techniques

Since they cannot hear the sound of the cane touching the surface of the ground, many deaf-blind travelers prefer to glide the tip along the surface so they gain more information about the texture of the ground or floor. This constant-contact technique can be tricky outdoors, where the cane tip is likely to get stuck in every crack, but people have been able to master a smooth movement, even with the chalk-shaped nylon tips. Mobility instructor Barbara Seever noted that some people who find the constant-contact technique awkward prefer to use the touch-and-slide cane technique. Cane tips that glide more easily are marshmallow tips, tips shaped like mushrooms or teardrops, rolling tips, and ball tips. The deaf-blind person can try various tips to see which gives him or her the most information about the surface.

Many people who are deaf-blind prefer to shoreline along the edge of sidewalks, rather than walk down the middle. At first, I discouraged them from this practice, since it is easy to veer into driveways if one follows the grass, and walking along the curb can be awkward because of poles and parking meters. Nevertheless, since it is harder for people who are deaf-blind to recognize whether they are on the sidewalk or in the street if they do not contact the edge of the sidewalk, they usually prefer to contend with poles and driveways than to walk down the middle of the sidewalk and take their chances on veering into the street. Thus, I now teach those who wish to do so how to walk along the edge with a minimum of veering into openings. I also make sure that they pay attention not only to the cane as they walk along, but to any inclines under their feet, so they can recognize and use slopes and gutters to identify the edge of the street as dependably as possible.

Some deaf-blind people also prefer a wider arc than normal, perhaps to get more information about their surroundings. However, when one uses the touch technique, a wider arc can be dangerous, since the farther to the side that the cane contacts the ground, the less warning the person has of drop-offs that are ahead. Therefore, when using a wide arc the constant-contact cane technique is preferable because the cane contacts the ground ahead as well as to each side. When descending stairs, many deaf-blind people, regardless of whether they have balance difficulties, prefer to use the cane to touch the edge of the next stair, rather than to hold the cane above the edge.

Even though they cannot hear the cane touching the ground, deaf-blind people are no more likely to have difficulty with the cane's rhythm than are hearing-blind people. However, many of my clients (both deaf and hearing) found it difficult at first to remain in rhythm when using the constant-contact cane technique even after they had established good rhythm with the touch technique. Mobility instructor Mary Michaud-Cooney found the opposite to be true: Her clients found it easier to stay in rhythm when using the constant-contact technique than the touch technique. If a person is having difficulty staying in rhythm with either technique, try teaching the other technique first. Once the rhythm is well established, allow the person to try again using the technique with which he or she was having difficulty.

When people are having difficulty with rhythm, whether they are hearing or deaf, I have found it effective to have them put down the cane and either pat their hip, move their hand back and forth, or clap in rhythm with their walk. While doing so, they walk using their vision or a sighted guide until they can easily move their hand in rhythm with their feet. Next they transfer this rhythm to the movement of the cane (either in the proper arc or, if this is too awkward at first, just tapping it on the ground in front of them).

Note: People should be cautioned to keep the cane tip on the ground (rather than use it as a pointer) and to fold and unfold it in such a manner that they will not stab others.

BALANCE*

Hearing people sometimes experience balance problems when they lose their vision, but people who are deaf, especially those with Usher's syndrome, Type I, experience balance problems more frequently. These problems concerned me greatly when I first

*This section was written in collaboration with Sandra Rosen, Ph.D., director, Program in Orientation and Mobility, San Francisco State University.

encountered them, but I found that in most cases, the balance problem diminishes as the person becomes more experienced walking with a loss of vision or working with a blindfold. Claes Möller (Möller, 1992), a Swedish otolaryngologist who specializes in balance, said that people with Usher's syndrome, Type I, "are born with few or no signals from their hearing or balance organs. They learn to walk late and may be clumsy at running games or sports. They learn to use their eyes and muscles, however, to improve their balance so they can walk and run normally. When they lose their vision . . . they feel unsteady again and become a little clumsy until they get used to their vision loss."

Balance is normally maintained by three senses: proprioception, vision, and the vestibular sense (Barr, 1974). *Proprioception* is the sense people use to maintain their balance while standing or walking; it informs them of the position of their body at each moment—the angles of joints, such as the ankles and legs, hip, neck, and shoulders. *Vision* augments proprioceptive information by enabling the person to align the body with vertical and horizontal lines in the environment. The *vestibular sense* is used most when a person loses his or her balance; it discerns the tilt of the head and recognizes when the head is upright again. The vestibular sense is most often affected in deaf people, since the mechanism for it (the semicircular canal) is housed in the inner ear.

When people who are visually impaired have difficulties with balance, usually their proprioception or their vestibular system is not functioning properly. The vestibular system can be impaired from birth, as often happens with people with Usher's syndrome. Other people experience impaired vestibular functioning later in life, sometimes with a loss of hearing and sometimes with their hearing intact.

The proprioceptive sense can be impaired by neurological problems, medications, or diabetic neuropathy (when it reduces a person's sensation of the movement and position of the ankles and feet). Also, people who are born totally blind and who do not receive early intervention do not fully develop their proprioceptive sense because they did not have the visual feedback normally used to develop it when they explored and manipulated their bodies as infants and young children. These people may have slightly impaired balance throughout life, for which they instinctively learn to compensate by using a different gait pattern, such as a wide base of support. Some components of gait patterns are mentioned later in this section.

Because proprioception and vision are the primary senses for balance while walking, people with normal vision may not notice an impairment of the vestibular system. However, when they lose vision they rely primarily on proprioception and may experience problems with their balance. Similarly, some people with normal vision automatically compensate for their impaired proprioception with vision and are oblivious to the impairment until they lose their sight.

Often these people assume that the balance problem was a consequence of the vision loss and are not aware that their vestibular or proprioceptive functioning was already deficient. These people may need to be referred to a physician, especially if they have any symptoms (such as difficulties in coordination, weak muscle groups, or sensory loss) that indicate a neurological problem. The physician may be able to determine whether the condition is stable or deteriorating and if intervention can correct or improve it.

Coping with Balance Difficulties

Most of my clients with impaired vestibular systems improved their proprioceptive sense naturally while walking. In general, remaining active is important for developing and preserving the use of the proprioceptive sense, especially activities that require more reliance on proprioception. These activities include walking on uneven surfaces and balance beams, as well as ice skating and skiing, which train ankles to be rigid and create more signals to the brain to maintain the upright position (skiing also enlarges the area of the foot's contact with the ground, emphasizing the proprioceptive signals). Laura Engler, who has Usher's syndrome, suggests walking on surfaces like grass, uneven pavement, and sand. Physical therapist Diane Ignatius suggests leaning slightly off balance and straightening up again. You can also gently push the person's shoulders to the side, back, or front to let him or her feel the tilt and straighten up again. Another good exercise is for the person to stand straight while holding one leg off the ground (and avoid leaning excessively toward the side on which he or she is standing).

All these activities can help fine-tune the proprioceptive sense, so it can maintain equilibrium. Since good muscle tone is essential for the proprioceptive sense, resistive exercises, such as swimming or moving in water, are also beneficial. Bicycling can be difficult for a person with an impaired vestibular system; it may be best to bicycle in tandem with a companion who has no problem with balance.

People who have learned to compensate for balance difficulties develop a gait with which they can walk more steadily. Often it includes taking smaller steps, with toes facing more toward the side, and a wider stance, with the feet sometimes almost as wide apart as the width of their bodies. If the stance is too wide, however, it can interfere with the efficiency of the gait and the fluidity of the person's movement.

On stairs, people with precarious balance use a handrail, when possible, although they may practice using no rail to be sure they can do so. Many also use the cane to contact each stair when going down, either touching the cane's tip on the top of the next stair or reaching beyond the edge of the next stair and dropping the cane down to contact the edge. Some people like to use the cane for a little support when there is no handrail or on curbs, but they should be cautious about doing so because the cane may slip while their weight is on it. If the person really needs support on stairs, a support cane is recommended. This cane should be measured by a physical therapist or at certain orthopedic-supply stores.

At both curbs and stairs, it is important that people with balance difficulties use the proper techniques. Some people stand with their back leg too far from the edge when their other leg reaches forward to step up or down. It is usually more stable to stand with one foot solidly at the edge before stepping up or down with the other foot. When standing for a while at the edge of a drop-off, people may lose the sensation of the edge under their feet; to regain it, mobility instructor and AFB national program associate Elga Joffee suggested that they wiggle their toes when they are ready to step down, to feel exactly where the edge is. Of course, the person's posture should be such that the center of gravity is forward when going up and on the heels when going down.

When using a sighted guide, people with balance difficulties may prefer to hook their arm around the guide's bent arm to use the guide for some support as well as guidance. Another grip, suggested by mobility instructor Barbara Seever for short distances, is for the deaf-blind person to reach inside the guide's arm to grasp the wrist, leaning the forearm on the guide's hip when descending stairs or curbs. Give people feedback as to how comfortable or fatiguing it is for you to support them. Those who need a lot of support may need to use only guides who are strong enough to provide it.

Some people with balance difficulties walk behind the guide and hold his or her shoulders for support. This technique is not recommended because the guide is vulnerable to being pulled off balance (perhaps being injured from the unexpected wrenching), the guide's ability to give the deaf-blind person information (about a narrow passage, for example) is reduced, and the guide is less able to assist if the deaf-blind person starts to lose his or her grip.

Occasionally I have worked with people who have a moderate balance problem but who use the guide for more support than is necessary. In some cases, they may do so because their balance and stability fluctuate. However, if the person seems consistently able to keep upright when walking alone, but maintains his or her balance by hanging and pulling on you while you are guiding, inform him or her how exhausting it is. If he or she continues to do so, discuss it and try letting your arm go limp, without supporting the person. This gesture can remind and encourage the person to use you for guidance, not to lean and hang on.

I developed this strategy out of necessity when guiding a deaf visually impaired man for several days. The man was able to walk unassisted without a support cane (although he staggered somewhat), but he pulled and leaned excessively while being guided. I held my arm stiffly to offer support but eventually my knee was badly wrenched, and for several days I tried to keep my weight off that leg. To my surprise, when I stopped holding my arm stiffly to support the man, he used my arm for guidance without hanging on me.

A few people with whom I worked (usually those who were frail or elderly) needed a support cane in addition to the white cane. I find that many people (hearing as well as deaf) do not know the different purposes of the two canes (especially since some of the support canes are painted white). I carefully explain that the purpose of the support cane is to support, and the purpose of the long white cane (which I sometimes call the "probing cane" or a "bumper") is to probe ahead. I then emphasize that one cane cannot perform both functions—when reaching forward with a cane to probe, one cannot use it for support, and while holding it close and leaning on a cane, one cannot use it to probe ahead. If a person needs both support and a probe, he or she needs two canes. Such clients practice walking in step and rhythm with both canes and usually become skilled and comfortable using both at the same time.

Some elderly hearing people with whom I worked did not need support, but they believed that when they lost some of their vision, they needed a cane, which they assumed was a support cane. They learned to use and depend on a white support cane. After I taught them how to use a long cane to probe, they concluded that they did not need a support cane after all. However, according to mobility instructor and AFB national program associate Elga Joffee, it can be difficult for some people to adjust to not using a support cane because they had readjusted their sensory integration for balance when they started to use it.

Traveling in a Wheelchair or Scooter

Sometimes clients require a wheelchair because their vestibular systems have been destroyed by surgery and they have no way of knowing if their bodies are vertical or horizontal. Others need a wheelchair or scooter because of physical disabilities, such as arthritis or a stroke.

Deaf-blind people who are motivated can travel independently in a wheelchair. One totally blind woman with a moderate hearing loss in one ear and no hearing in the other travels with her wheelchair independently to work and meetings by taxis and travels alone throughout the country. (She finds that holding a folded $5 bill in her hand when she arrives at an airport terminal usually guarantees that someone will approach her quickly to offer assistance.) Another totally blind man with a moderate hearing loss and decreased motor function from a stroke can travel independently from his apartment to shopping nearby (getting assistance to cross the street because he cannot hear the cars well enough). Many deaf-blind people who travel in wheelchairs are developmentally disabled and may not be able to travel in unfamiliar environments, but are able to learn to travel independently in familiar settings.

The instructor can help the motivated wheelchair user who is deaf-blind learn many of the same skills that other visually impaired people learn, to achieve the level of independent travel that they desire and have the potential to attain. These skills include how to judge distances and turns, move forward with a minimum of veering (for example, learning to move each wheel a consistent amount to go straight), use spatial memory and touch to remain oriented, solicit aid, communicate with salespeople, and use taxis or public transportation.

Visually impaired wheelchair users often travel independently in familiar settings (such as their home or work) without a cane. Those who travel in unfamiliar areas, near stairs, or in uncontrolled environments in a wheelchair can use a white cane in conjunction with the wheelchair. Suggest to the client and his or her physical therapist that they consider a wheelchair in which the client can have a hand free to use a cane. Some wheelchairs are designed to be used with one hand (the wheels can be locked so that moving one wheel propels both wheels). People who use a wheelchair because of balance difficulties often can use their legs to pull the chair forward. Ask the physical therapist if this would be feasible for your client, because it leaves both hands free.

Nurion Industries manufactures two electronic travel aids that can be adapted to provide hands-free tactile output for those who do not have a hand free to use a cane or who want the security and information that electronic travel aids can provide. The Wheelchair Pathfinder can be attached to wheelchairs and walkers to detect obstacles as far as eight feet ahead and most drop-offs. The Polaron, which provides tactile output as well, can be hung around the neck to detect obstacles (it will not detect drop-offs).

USE OF THE REMAINING SENSES

The sensory information received by totally blind, profoundly deaf travelers is severely restricted because they lack the two senses that most efficiently provide distance information. As a result, the world of the deaf-blind person is often described as not extending "beyond the reach of his or her hands and feet."

This phrase helps convey to lay people the importance of contacting the deaf-blind person for communication. It helps them appreciate how insulated the person's world can be (see Chapter 5) and emphasizes that the deaf-blind person will usually not be aware of what occurs nearby unless he or she is told.

However, the phrase also conveys the misconception that people who are deaf-blind do not know what is beyond their reach. In fact, deaf-blind people can use their spatial memory and kinesthetic and tactile senses to know where they are, what is around them, and where their objective is. For example, while driving a deaf-blind man to our lesson, I missed our turn. I thought of this phrase and smiled when he stopped talking and said, "Haven't you gone too far? You were supposed to turn left before the top of the hill."

The deaf-blind traveler can develop and rely on these senses and spatial memory for steady information but can also use occasional information, such as vibrations, air movement, temperature changes, and odors. During a 1985 hearing of the U.S. Department of Transportation, Robert J. Smithdas, assistant director, Helen Keller

National Center for Deaf-Blind Youths and Adults, stated that he would know if the plane in which he was riding crash-landed because he would feel the deceleration and jolt. If there were a fire, he would smell smoke, and he would know if he was near the fire by its heat. If he felt fresh air, he would know there was an opening to the outside, and by feeling people rushing down the aisle by his seat, he would know which way the people were going. Thus, although deaf-blind people's information about their surroundings is severely restricted, it is no more accurate to say that their world does not extend beyond their hands and feet than it would be to say the same thing about blind people. Excellent descriptions of the use of the remaining senses can be found in Kinney (1972, pp. 1–8) and Michaud (1990).

Kinesthetic and Tactile Senses

When alone in a quiet, familiar room, people with an intact spatial memory who are hearing-blind or deaf-blind are relatively certain where the furniture and doors are, without reaching out to touch them. With practice, they can move with equal ease around the room. The predominant senses that they would use are the kinesthetic sense and the tactile sense. The kinesthetic sense helps them judge how far to walk and how much to turn to reach the objective or get around an obstacle, and the tactile sense can help them verify where they are as they come in contact with and identify features in the room. The blind person who can hear may also verify information with echolocation and the sound of his or her body or cane touching surfaces. If the person was deprived of this auditory information, however, he or she could still be well oriented.

When traveling outside, the hearing-blind person can use additional auditory information for orientation. However, the deaf-blind person can still use his or her spatial memory and kinesthetic and tactile senses to know where he is in relation to the buildings, streets, and curbs. With efficient use of a cane or a dog, he or she can travel confidently.

Vibration, Air Movement, and Temperature

Movements and sounds cause the surrounding air and objects to vibrate. If the sound or movement is loud or strong enough, you can feel the vibration in your body. Lesser vibrations can be felt when you touch an object that is vibrating. If the object is vibrating because of something that is touching it, you can sometimes determine the direction of the source of vibration, especially if the surface of the object is large and you place both hands or both feet apart on the object. For example, when standing on a wooden floor, people who are deaf-blind can often determine the direction of people who are walking nearby. While occluding your eyes and ears, place your hands apart on a table, and you should be able to tell approximately where someone else is knocking on the table. Some people can detect the presence of heavy nearby traffic and other loud environmental sounds by feeling the vibrations in an inflated balloon, an umbrella, or another object.

The deaf-blind person can often detect landmarks, such as doorways, windows, and the edges of buildings, by the air moving through or around them and by the change in temperature of the air that is coming through a window or a door. They can also feel moving air as people, cars, or trains pass by and determine their orientation using the sun.

Developing the Use of Remaining Senses

In general, I teach deaf-blind people how to use their remaining senses in the same manner that I use with hearing-blind people. With some people, especially those whose vision fluctuates, I use a blindfold or partial occlusion occasionally to increase their sensory awareness and to promote an understanding of how to use techniques without vision.

Some professionals say that blindfolds should not be used when teaching deaf visually impaired people because their fear of blindness is too great. I have not found this to be true. When I use blindfolds and partial occlusion during training, I have found that deaf visually impaired people are as willing to use them and benefit as greatly from the experience as do hearing people.

However, when deaf people who rely on vision cannot see, communication is limited. Thus, the discussion of what to expect and on what sensory input to concentrate needs to take place before they put on blindfolds. Also, the blindfold experience should occur after they have mastered the technique being used. For example, before I ask clients to walk blindfolded with me to increase their awareness of sensory information, I make sure they are comfortable using a sighted guide without a blindfold. I then find out what they are willing to try with a blindfold. As always, whether teaching clients who are blindfolded or clients who are blind, I gauge how challenging to make the experience (how many turns or doors or stairs to use) by how comfortable or frightened they are with the experience. They take off the blindfold afterward to discuss it. Likewise, I do not ask clients to walk alone wearing a blindfold in unfamiliar areas until they are comfortable with and skilled in using a cane.

Vision

Primary among the senses to be assessed and utilized is any remaining vision, which is even more important for a deaf person than for a hearing person. Even a small field of vision, for instance, can enable some deaf clients to cross certain busy streets safely if they learn to use that vision efficiently.

I usually assess and develop the visual functioning of deaf and hearing clients in the same way. Every client should understand how lighting affects his or her vision and how to maximize the use of that vision. For those with a central or peripheral visual loss, I explain that the central visual system detects details and color and the peripheral visual system detects movement and contrast. I then teach techniques for utilizing the strengths of their remaining visual system (central or peripheral) to make up for the loss of the other system. Eccentric viewing for people who have lost their central vision and scanning and tracking methods for those with restricted visual fields are two such techniques. A functional curriculum for assessing the vision and hearing of deaf-blind adults was developed by the Canadian National Institute for the Blind (CNIB, 1992) (see Resources).

Sometimes when deaf people with restricted visual fields search for me, their eyes dart from side to side but miss me. They can no longer find things by glancing quickly like they did when they had usable peripheral vision because the central visual system cannot discern details of rapid movement as well as the peripheral visual system can. When they search more slowly, they are usually able to find me with the first scan. This skill can be applied to many situations, including looking for cars when crossing the street (see "Crossing Intersections With No Traffic Light" in Chapter 8). This slow scanning is not necessary unless the visual field is severely restricted; help your client assess whether he or she needs to scan slowly or can still locate things efficiently by glancing.

Hearing

Any residual hearing should also be assessed for the ability to identify and localize sounds and to echolocate (see De L'Aune, 1980; Wiener, 1980; and CNIB, 1992 for information on assessing and developing remaining hearing). Localization can be enhanced by cupping the ears with the hands and then moving the head. With a unilateral or asymmetrical hearing loss, localization can be improved by moving the head. The person can try different methods of head movement (such as fast, slow, or to one side) until he or she finds the most efficient ways to move the head to localize different sounds. The ability to localize may also be developed to some degree by people with limited hearing if they learn to recognize when a sound gets louder or softer as they approach or walk away from the source.

Even though echolocation is based on hearing, it is worthwhile to determine if the hearing-impaired person can develop this ability. According to Wiener (1980), echolocation is based on the ability to detect differences in the pitch of sounds primarily of frequencies between 10,000 and 12,000 Hz. Auditory ability above 8,000 Hz is not usually measured by audiologists, and some people have useful hearing in that frequency that has not been documented. A few of my hard-of-hearing clients could use echolocation to some degree, and one deaf client whose hearing loss was predominantly below 8,000 Hz was able to echolocate in certain circumstances.

To test the potential for echolocation, I usually use a concave item, such as a bowl or mold, that reflects sound into a more concentrated area than does a flat object. When the client can tell when the bowl is near the ear, I know he or she has some ability to echolocate and I help him or her to develop the use of that ability in the environment.

People who think that they may have lost some hearing when they lost their vision should have their hearing tested. Sometimes, those with a slight hearing loss are not aware that they relied on lipreading to understand people until they lose their vision. Conversely, some people with normal hearing who, like most people, unconsciously lipread in noisy environments, mistakenly think they have lost some hearing when they can no longer see the faces of those who are speaking.

The instructor should be aware that many audiologists are not experienced with hearing-impaired people who are blind and that their primary concern is their patients' ability to hear speech, which is at frequencies of 500–2,000 Hz. The audiologist who is fitting hearing aids for the deaf visually impaired person needs to consider that the person may benefit from aids or amplifiers that can improve the ability to hear environmental sounds at frequencies above and below those required for speech. Echolocation requires the ability to hear 10,000–12,000 Hz (Wiener, 1980), and although the sound of traffic covers the entire audible frequency range of 20–20,000 Hz, the most intense sounds are at the lower frequencies. Wiener measured traffic sounds in business and residential areas and found that at a frequency of 125 Hz, the loudness of the traffic is 69–78 Db, but at 12,500 Hz, the intensity is only half that amount.

For those who cannot detect environmental sounds, vibrotactile devices can transform sounds into vibrations (see Resources). Vibrotactile devices can help deaf-blind travelers recognize if they are walking along a quiet residential street or a busy urban street, detect voices and footsteps of people nearby, and identify when a bus approaches. With these devices, the person can learn to distinguish many sounds by their duration, intensity, and rhythm (for example, to differentiate a knock on the door from a passing fire truck). Vibrotactile devices that have more than one channel, each of which responds to a certain frequency range, allow the user to recognize some sounds by their frequencies as well (for example, to distinguish the sound of running water from that of a distant train). The more channels the device has, the more information the user will have to distinguish sounds.

Olfactory Sense

Some people think that the sense of smell is the predominant sense of deaf-blind travelers. However, as Michaud (1990, p. 148) noted, "The olfactory system is often too unreliable to be used as a primary sensory input system, but it can be used to back up [information from the other senses]."

The deaf-blind person, like the hearing-blind person, can identify some places by unique odors, as well as people who use a favorite fragrance or who smoke certain brands of cigarettes. However, it is a myth that deaf-blind people can recognize most individuals by their odor.

Kinesthetic Sense and Spatial Memory

Until I worked with my first deaf-blind client, I thought that hearing was the most important sense for the blind traveler. After working with people who are deaf-blind, I realized that at least in quiet, familiar areas, hearing-blind travelers, like deaf-blind travelers, mainly use the kinesthetic and tactile senses. Thus, although I still teach hearing clients how to maximize the use of their hearing, I now emphasize the development of the kinesthetic and tactile senses with both hearing-blind and deaf-blind clients.

Early in the mobility program for both deaf and hearing blind clients who cannot rely on visual information to remain oriented, I assess clients' ability to walk without vision accurately and with confidence through areas with which they are familiar. If improvement is needed, they practice estimating turns and distances (both for short distances indoors and long distances outside). Exercises can include reestablishing the line of direction after walking around an obstacle and walking through a familiar obstacle course touching the obstacles as little as possible. Another helpful exercise is to guide the person along a twisted route (it could be in one room or throughout the building) to an objective and then to return to the starting point. The client then shows where he or she thinks the objective was. Clients with vision could use a blindfold while being guided.

ADDITIONAL CONSIDERATIONS

Confidentiality

Every person is entitled to privacy, but privacy is difficult to achieve when others are needed to help read one's mail, shop, bank, and visit a physician. One advantage of achieving independent mobility is gaining the ability to go places and do things without always involving others. If Helen Keller had been able to travel independently, perhaps it would have been easier for her to carry out her decisions and more difficult for others to thwart her plans (see Chapter 6).

During mobility training, however, the client's feelings of being patronized can inadvertently be fostered when the mobility instructor reports his or her progress to others without permission. Once when chatting with a client's son, I mentioned with pride that she had gone to the store and bought some cigarettes independently during her lesson. I did not realize that she had not told her family she had resumed smoking. For this client, being able to get to the store meant being able to buy the cigarettes without her being admonished by her family. Although it is important to include the client's family and other service providers in the rehabilitation process, it is equally important to do so only with the client's permission and knowledge.

Another factor to consider is that the deaf and the deaf-blind communities are small. Because they each have a common language that is not shared with the general population, both communities are more closely knit than are most other communities, including the blind community. I routinely refrain from discussing a client's progress with other clients because even if no names are mentioned, it does not take long to figure out whom I might be talking about. When they make a mistake, some clients remark that they wonder what so-and-so will say about it, apparently assuming that the person will inevitably learn about it. I assure them that reports of their progress are not shared with others without their permission.

Duration of Training

In some cases, the client cannot communicate while he or she is doing something else. The easy interaction I can have with hearing clients as we walk or drive to a lesson and my verbal explanations while they proceed with the lesson must be done before or after the activity or lesson with many deaf-blind clients. In other cases, communication between the instructor and deaf-blind client is slower than it is with a hearing client.

In these situations, the duration of training is often longer than it is for a hearing client. For example, lessons that required only one hour for most hearing clients required three hours for several of my deaf-blind clients with whom communication was slow. It took an hour to prepare them for the route, another hour for them to complete the route, and a third hour to discuss all that happened and plan how to improve it the next time.

Distance of the Instructor from the Client

Many deaf-blind clients must be touched to get their attention and communicate with them. Some instructors conclude that since it is not possible to give these clients verbal warnings, they should keep within arm's distance of the clients at all times during training. If they do so, however, they cannot step back and observe deaf-blind clients unobtrusively while they travel independently.

It is at least as important for the deaf-blind client to practice traveling independently while the instructor observes from a distance as it is for the hearing client (see "Role of the Instructor" in Chapter 4). We need to consider, then, whether the instructor should allow deaf-blind clients to travel out of arm's reach, as is done with hearing-blind clients.

The apparent reason that some professionals think that the instructor should be within arm's reach of deaf-blind clients but not of hearing-blind clients is that they feel assured that hearing clients will respond to verbal warnings. However, this may not necessarily be true, as illustrated by the following examples:

- In 1985, I attended a hearing of the U.S. Department of Transportation. An airline company claimed that deaf-blind travelers should be denied permission to travel alone on airplanes because they would not be able to respond to verbal commands during an emergency. I heard a witness for the airline admit, however, that during emergencies some nondisabled people are also unable to respond to verbal commands, possibly because they are immobilized with fear.

- According to Elga Joffee, mobility instructor and AFB national program associate, many people are "temporarily sensory impaired" because of such environmental conditions as noise, smog, and obstacles. Thus, when clients who have normal hearing are near a noisy intersection, they may not be able to heed verbal warnings because they cannot hear them.
- Many blind travelers become accustomed to and may ignore strangers calling out unnecessary warnings when they are headed toward a pole or another "danger."

Mobility instructors should realize, then, that a client (whether hearing or deaf) may not always respond appropriately when they shout directions or warnings because the client cannot hear the warning, is not paying attention because he or she is concentrating on something else, does not realize that the instructor is issuing the warning, or hears but is unable to respond because he or she was startled or afraid.

Therefore, the instructor should try to anticipate problems as much as possible and be nearby when the client (hearing or deaf) may do something unsafe. As Lolli (1980, p. 444) suggested, the instructor should be within quick reach of the deaf-blind client especially "in the beginning phases of instruction when both parties are becoming familiar with one another's communication skills and it is an easy time for discrepancies to occur"; during these phases of training, the instructor learns what to expect from the client and how reliably he or she uses safe techniques. Of course, no client is ever totally predictable, but the instructor should strive to anticipate danger as much as possible.

When the client has demonstrated the reliable use of safe techniques, the instructor and client should discuss how far away the instructor will be when the client is traveling. The client should know that the instructor may not be nearby if he or she makes a mistake, would find it awkward or confusing if he or she thought the instructor was nearby when a stranger approached, and may lose trust if the instructor is not where the client thought he or she was. If the client and instructor agree that the client can safely travel the route or parts of it, the instructor can drop back and observe from a distance far enough to allow the public to interact and far enough for the client to have a sense of traveling independently while being observed. If something happens to cause the instructor to question whether the client will perform safely, the instructor then moves closer.

It is vital that the deaf-blind traveler be allowed to interact with the public alone (see "Role of the Instructor" in Chapter 4). Thus when the instructor must remain close, he or she uses every subterfuge available to remain anonymous, just as is done with hearing-blind clients. Like most mobility instructors, I have waited nearby at countless bus stops, pretended to make calls at nearby telephone booths, done a lifetime of window shopping, and often stopped to check the contents of my pockets or readjust my watch.

To signal the client from a distance, the instructor may use a vibrating device that the client carries in a pocket and that the instructor activates with a remote control. The device could be made inexpensively using the equipment from a remote-control toy car, with the receiver and motor encased in such a way that the motor vibrates the framework and the car's remote control acts as the transmitter. Or, a pager, or vibrating alerting system, such as Silent Call's Omni Page Receiver and transmitter can be purchased (see Resources). Such a device would have come in handy when I had to run after deaf clients to give them different instructions or new information! Perhaps the instructor and the client could set up a series of signals ("beep" could mean "Your arc is narrow again"; "beep-beep" could mean "Don't forget to keep your head up—your posture is starting to sag"; and "beeeeep" could mean "Wait; I have something to tell you"). However, when one client and I tried using a pager so I could get his attention, he did not react to it consistently. Thus, although a remote-control vibrating device may be helpful for communication, you should *not* rely on it to warn deaf-blind clients of danger, just as shouting should not be relied upon to warn hearing clients.

Electronic Travel Aids

Since the two most efficient distance senses of people who are deaf-blind are impaired, it would seem that they would benefit greatly from electronic travel aids (ETAs) (see Glossary). ETAs that provide tactile output and can therefore be used by people who are deaf-blind are the Mowat Sensor, the Polaron, the laser cane, the Wheelchair Pathfinder, and the Pathsounder (see Resources). The Polaron and the Pathsounder can be either hand held or hung on the chest for hands-free use. (For a discussion of the Wheelchair Pathsounder, see "Traveling in a Wheelchair or Scooter" earlier in this chapter).

Although these ETAs would seem ideally suited for deaf-blind travelers, it has been my experience that few people who are deaf-blind use them. Michaud (1990) reported that in her survey of 154 deaf-blind users of mass transit, only 8 used an ETA (the Mowat Sensor). Some of these travelers were not considered appropriate users of the Mowat Sensor because they had remaining vision or were mentally retarded. Others said that they did not use it because it needed to be maintained and recharged and that the information it provided "was superfluous because [the travelers] were familiar with the route they were using and the landmarks. Others felt they already had enough to carry, such as a cane, communication cards, writing guides, and tactile maps. Still others objected to the constant vibration from the device, which was caused by the presence of many people on the [mass transit] platform or at the bus stop" (Michaud, 1990, pp. 148–149).

Although few people who are deaf-blind use ETAs, their advantages as a mobility device, Michaud (1990) concluded, "are reason enough to make [their] use an important option in O&M training." ETAs are useful for finding landmarks and overhangs and paths through the woods and for locating pedestrians to solicit aid or to recognize when a bus arrives. Instructors should make sure that their clients are aware of the advantages of ETAs and have the opportunity to try them.

Other electronic devices may also help deaf-blind travelers (see "Electronic Devices" in Chapter 8). Vibrotactile devices (see Glossary), such as TACTAID II+ (see Resources), enable deaf people to detect sounds in the environment, including footsteps, voices, nearby traffic, and even birds, with the vibration of the receptors placed on the wrist or chest. Although these devices do not provide enough information to detect cars for street crossings, they can help the deaf-blind traveler be aware of such environmental sounds as a busy street, pedestrians, or an approaching bus.

Footwear

What to wear on the feet is a dilemma. On the one hand, it is good to have shoes with soles that are thin enough to feel the ground surface more easily. On the other hand, blind people who cannot hear the objects that the cane hits are more vulnerable to stepping on broken glass or other sharp objects, from which thicker soles may protect them. Indoors, many deaf-blind people routinely wear protective footwear because they are not always aware when glass has been knocked off a counter or table onto the floor.

SPECIFIC SITUATIONS

Shopping

Except for the communication method used, shopping skills for deaf-blind travelers are almost identical to those for hearing-blind travelers. In most instances, it is best to shop when the store is not busy. When a person cannot see well enough to find and select merchandise, he or she approaches the counter or manager's office to get assistance. If the store is unfamiliar and the person does not know where the counter is, he or she can enter and solicit aid using a card, voice, or other communication method. (See Figures 2A and B.) At grocery stores, some deaf-blind people give their shopping lists to the store personnel and wait until the personnel return with the items to buy, and others go with the personnel to select items and take advantage of sales.

It is best to learn to shop by first trying it in relatively structured settings, such as small shops, dry cleaners, fast-food restaurants, and post offices, where one's communication needs can be anticipated. The purpose of the visit is self-evident, the counter is usually easy to find, and one can anticipate the information that the clerk will probably request and answer.

Deaf-blind people who are learning to shop in their own communities usually go to the stores beforehand and introduce themselves to let the salespeople know how to communicate with them. Some people prefer that an interpreter or instructor accompany them, which often makes the introduction go more smoothly. However, it is important that deaf-blind people also learn to introduce themselves and establish communication independently.

If you or an interpreter will accompany the deaf-blind person for this introduction, it is the deaf-blind person who should make the introduction (through an interpreter, if desired) and explain to the salesperson how to communicate, rather than be passively introduced. Describe the situation to the deaf-blind person beforehand and role-play if necessary. Also discuss how he or she wants the interpretation to be handled. Sometimes when I interpret by signing or fingerspelling, salespeople are astonished and intimidated and are reluctant to try to communicate themselves. Thus, I sometimes interpret by using the method of communication that the salesperson will need to use (such as print on palm or writing notes). If the situation is hectic or awkward and it is more important that the communication go smoothly, it may be best to interpret with whatever method is most proficient, such as sign language or fingerspelling. As always while you are interpreting for people who are deaf-blind, inform your client of what is happening, so he or she can gauge how to respond (is the salesperson frowning and quiet, distracted by the phone or other customers, or smiling and leaning forward, eager to communicate?)

Once people who are deaf-blind become comfortable shopping, it is often hard for them to realize that even though they know the personnel at a store, they will still sometimes find salespeople who do not realize that they are deaf or who do not know them. The friendly manager at the grocery store may be temporarily replaced with a substitute, and the small shop where everyone is familiar may have a new employee alone at the store. It is important that deaf-blind people be able to recognize when the situation has changed and to then establish communication assuming that they may be dealing with a stranger. For example, a deaf-blind man who was familiar with the grocery store personnel was stopped by someone as he entered the store. He assumed

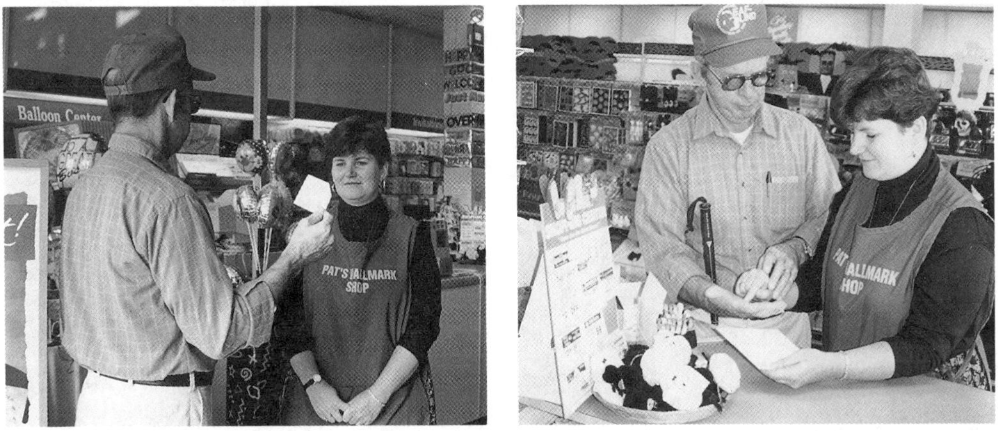

Figures 2A and B. This deaf-blind shopper uses a card to find a salesperson. The salesperson helps him select greeting cards by printing on his palm. By placing his hand on hers as she prints, he can more easily identify the letters.

that the person knew him and was perplexed that she did not explain to him why she stopped him. After a long wait, he went around her and continued on his way. He later found out that this salesperson had set up a table for free samples and that she did not know him or realize that he was deaf. When he did not respond to her instructions to get around her table, she just blocked his way.

Some salespeople are flustered or do not want to bother to communicate with the deaf-blind customer. They may just ignore the customer or substitute another item without explaining if they do not have what the customer wants. The person who is deaf-blind may need to explain (by note or voice) how the salespeople can indicate that they are too busy to help and that he or she should wait until they have the time to communicate or until they can page someone who can help ("Please tap my hand three times if I will need to wait for service.").

With these interactions, it is helpful if the instructor can inconspicuously observe and later report to the client what happened. For example, what was the apparent attitude of the salespeople, and what was happening while the client waited? If necessary, the instructor and deaf-blind person can brainstorm to figure out ways to improve the situation.

Using Public Transportation

People who are deaf-blind travel independently in carpools, paratransit systems, taxis, buses, subways, trains, and airplanes. They use many of the same techniques as do hearing-blind people. Each traveler will decide how much assistance he or she will need for each route and how to get that assistance (see Michaud, 1990, for helpful information about using public transportation).

To use any transportation system successfully requires good communication skills, careful planning, and knowledge of how to use that system. With buses, one must know how to call for route information, how to find the door and the fare box, and seating arrangements; with taxis and paratransit systems, one must know how to arrange a ride and payment policies; with subways, one must know how to use tokens or farecards and to enter the gates, the arrangement of the platforms and subway cars, and where the station attendants can be found; and with airplanes, one must know baggage check-in procedures, how to find the gate or assistance to get to it, how to use the buttons in the passenger seat, where the emergency exits are, and how to put on the life jacket and oxygen mask.

Buses

Most people who are deaf-blind can use their remaining vision or hearing or an ETA to determine when a bus arrives. If they cannot reliably detect the arrival of a bus, they need to use a card, voice, or tape recording to ask others to inform them when the bus arrives. Voice and tape should be used only when there are many people nearby; if alone, the deaf-blind person will need to use a card that is large enough for the bus driver to read. (See "Initiating Communication or Soliciting Aid" in Chapter 3 for ideas.) The card could contain the following information:

1. At the top: "BUS" in large letters or the name or number of the desired bus.

2. Next, in letters large enough for the bus driver to see after pulling up: "Please *TAP ME* when the bus arrives. I am *DEAF* and *BLIND*."

3. At the bottom in smaller print: "You can print letters in my palm with your finger."

In Seattle, the bus company distributes a folding plastic sign, with see-through pockets into which the traveler places the number of the desired bus. The driver stops when he sees a person holding up the number of his bus, and he can tell by the color of the cards whether the passenger is blind or deaf-blind.

When the bus arrives and the deaf-blind person cannot detect its arrival, others who are waiting for the bus and who read the card or heard the request for assistance will usually guide him or her to it. If the deaf-blind person is standing alone and people in the bus can easily read his or her card, the driver or another passenger will often get out to guide him or her to the door. The person then uses a prepared communication method to verify that it is the right bus. Some people use voice or a note to ask the driver to tap a yes-no signal while they hold out their hand ("Please tap me twice if this is the 34 bus to Argonne Street, since I cannot hear or see you"), and others who have some vision ask drivers to shake their head yes or no. If they use speech, it may help to sign while speaking, so the driver and passengers realize that they are deaf. It is also wise for deaf-blind people to inform the driver how to communicate with them, since sometimes after they have sat down, drivers have tried to tell them that they are on the wrong bus or that they gave the incorrect fare.

If the person needs assistance to know when the bus arrives at the right stop, before sitting down he or she should hand the driver a note or card (see Figure 3).The wording on the card can help prevent such problems as the driver forgetting the person's stop and asking again or announcing the person's stop verbally even after being informed that the person is deaf-blind. If the drivers keep these notes or cards, they can refer to them if they forget which stop the deaf-blind person wants, and it is less likely that they will forget to announce the stop. Even if a driver announces the person's stop verbally, the traveler can be alerted that it is time to disembark when the driver hands him or her the card or asks another passenger to do so. Also, some dri-

Please KEEP this card and
RETURN it to me when we
arrive at
K Street and 20th.

I am DEAF and BLIND.
You can print letters on my
palm with your finger.
THANK YOU!

Figure 3. A sample card for use during travel.

vers have alerted deaf-blind people that they are on the wrong bus when they saw the name of the destination on the note.

Mobility instructor Mary Michaud-Cooney suggested that to help drivers remember to announce the stop, visually impaired travelers can sit near the door, across the aisle from the driver so the driver sees them every time he or she looks at passengers coming in the door. They may also hold in their lap a second card that indicates where they want to get off. This way, other passengers may remember to inform them, and if a new driver takes over (or the first driver forgets which passenger gave him or her the card), the second card can remind the driver who needs to be informed of the stop.

Using buses can be frustrating, but good preparation can alleviate most of the difficulties. Nevertheless, sometimes the bus will pass people by, or the driver will forget to announce a stop or will let a passenger off at the wrong stop. Although most visually impaired passengers experience these problems, the communication barrier adds to the difficulty for those who are also deaf. Drivers who let them off at the wrong stop may not inform them (or may not be aware that the person did not understand the explanation). When people talk to them or steer them toward a seat, the deaf-blind travelers may not understand what the people are trying to do.

Thus, bus travel should be introduced only after the person is experienced and successful in communicating and interacting with people and can handle frustration and unexpected problems. Again, feedback about what the driver or passengers are trying to communicate may help the person understand their behavior better in the future. It may also relieve deaf-blind people (and their instructors!) to realize that after they become experienced with a particular bus route, they and the drivers and passengers may become familiar with each other, and although these problems will not disappear, they will occur less frequently.

Taxis

Deaf-blind travelers use their preferred methods of communication to call taxi services. Some use amplifiers to understand speech, people with TDDs (including TDDs with braille output) can use relay systems, and others use a signal system (see "Yes-No Signals" in Chapter 2) that they explain to the dispatcher. An example of how such a signal system is used is the following exchange: "I am deaf and blind. Please answer my questions either no, yes-yes, or I-don't-understand. Do you understand?"; "Yes-yes"; "Can a taxi pick me up at such-and-such address in the next 15 minutes?"; "No"; "In the next half hour?" "Yes-yes."

When the traveler arranges for the taxi to come, he or she must explain to the dispatcher exactly how the driver will announce that the taxi has arrived and, if appropriate, report his or her visual and hearing impairment ("I am deaf and cannot see well" or "I am deaf and blind"). Some people explain that they will be waiting in front of their home or at the entrance to their building and the driver must tap them (they might need to describe what they are wearing or explain that they will have a white cane). Others have alerting systems or enough hearing that they can recognize when the driver rings their doorbell or knocks on their door. Some wait with their hand or back touching the door to feel the knocking. Others ask that the driver call the dispatcher upon arrival and have the dispatcher telephone the traveler, who then goes outside to the taxi (this is a good way to verify that it is the taxi driver and not an imposter).

Once the driver arrives, travelers use their preferred methods of communication to verify that it is the driver, explain where they want to go, and describe how the driver can communicate to them. Some people who use voice also give the driver a note disclosing the destination and how to communicate, in case the driver doesn't understand or forgets their verbal explanation. Travelers should carefully explain (repeatedly if necessary) how the driver can communicate and inform them that they have reached the destination because even after careful explanations, drivers often do not realize that their passengers are deaf and cannot understand speech.

When they arrive, most drivers are willing to guide the person to the door of the building or office. The travelers may need to explain again how the driver can inform them of the fare.

Subway Systems

Although some travelers think that subways are frightening, others prefer them because once they are familiar with the route, little communication is needed. Of course, all travelers in subway systems, especially those whose vision is affected by the dim lighting in many stations, must have reliable mobility skills to avoid falling from the platforms. If deaf-blind travelers know how to find and communicate with station attendants and other people, they can get assistance or directions to travel in unfamiliar stations.

Most deaf-blind travelers cannot hear well enough to use the sound of people's movements for orientation, but they can use all the other techniques that hearing-blind travelers use to find the turnstiles or escalators, locate the door and enter the train, exit, and so forth. Once they are oriented on the platform, those who cannot see or hear the approaching trains can usually feel the train's air movement or vibrations. They may need to ask for assistance to identify which train it is if more than one train stops at their platform. Visually impaired travelers need to carefully check the floor before entering to be sure it is not the space between the cars. Once aboard, they can sit or stand near a door to count how many times it opens so they know when it has arrived at their station. They cannot rely on counting how many times the train stops, because sometimes the train stops between stations, but the doors remain closed. Once travelers are familiar with the route, they can recognize landmarks, such as which stations are close together and which are far apart or at which stations the doors open on the left and which on the right.

Using Elevators

A bank of elevators is one of the most aggravating aspects of indoor travel for some people who are deaf-blind. On the lobby floor, the person may be able to get assistance, but on upper floors or empty lobbies it is difficult to do so. Therefore, some people prefer to use stairs.

To get an elevator, the deaf-blind person can push the button, then stand between the elevator doors, with a hand touching one door and (if he or she can reach) with the cane touching the other. If there are more than two doors, he or she must repeatedly push the button because it will go off every time an elevator arrives at a door other than the two that the person is monitoring.

DEAF-BLIND PEOPLE AND DOG GUIDES*

Deaf-blind people use dog guides for many of the same reasons and in much the same manner as do hearing-blind people. Dog guides can enable them to travel smoothly around obstacles, quickly find doorways and landmarks with which they are familiar, and negotiate crowded areas. Both hearing-blind people and deaf-blind people must be well oriented and know where to direct their dogs to go. They must seek occasional assistance or directions when using their dog guides to find a new place or to reorient themselves when they become lost. Travelers who are deaf-blind may also need to seek assistance in other situations, such as at street crossings.

Primary Considerations

Dogs can learn to understand signals as well as verbal commands. Deaf people report that their pet dogs understand signed phrases, such as "Wanna go outside?" and "Stay!" In noisy places where it is difficult to understand verbal commands, dog guides of hearing-blind people often watch for signals so they know where to go. During obedience training, most dog guides learn the meaning of the words *sit, stay, come, down,* and *heel.* The deaf person who does not have understandable speech can teach the dog to understand signals for those commands.

Both deaf-blind and hearing-blind travelers can "feel" when their dogs have become distracted and need to be corrected. They can tell when the dogs turn their heads to look at something else or reach down to sniff. They can also note the dog's mood or emotions. For example, on a hot day Janice Adams can tell that her dog is feeling "blah" and walking slowly. On a new route, she sometimes notices her dog become excited and enthusiastic, walking briskly. Once her dog refused to go forward, and Janice noticed that the dog was shaking and was hunched up with her head down. Janice figured that she needed to watch out for something and reached forward

*This section was written in collaboration with Janice Adams, an instructor and consultant for organizations such as the Hearing-Visually Impaired Program at Gallaudet University. She is deaf-blind and uses a dog guide.

carefully with her foot to feel around. She found that they had come to the edge of a porch with no railing. When she realized why the dog was scared, she enthusiastically praised her for warning her of the danger.

Many people, including deaf-blind people and their families and those who work with them, assume that dog guides can do everything that human guides can do. The training of dogs to assist sighted deaf people is adding to the confusion. These "hearing ear dogs" wear an identifiable orange harness and leash and accompany their owners to alert them to such sounds as doorbells, telephones, and smoke and fire alarms. Many deaf people assume that a hearing ear dog can also serve as a dog guide for a person who is deaf-blind.

The instructor will usually need to dispel the myths and clarify how a dog guide for blind persons can be used. A dog guide cannot enable deaf-blind travelers to cross most streets independently or guide them to unfamiliar destinations. Chuck Farrugia of Guide Dogs for the Blind (see "Resources" at the back of this book for the addresses of the dog guide schools mentioned here) emphasizes that the traveler must be oriented well enough to give the appropriate commands to tell the dog guide where to go. Many dog guide schools will not accept applicants for dog guides who are unable to travel independently with a cane. As Ted Zubrycki of Guiding Eyes for the Blind said, "A person who travels poorly with a cane will not be made a better traveler through the use of a dog guide."

Dog Guide Schools and Training

Fifteen years ago, people who were deaf-blind were not accepted by most dog guide schools for several reasons. The schools believed that (1) deaf-blind students would not be able to communicate with their trainers, (2) trainers could not teach without being able to give students instructions from a distance to avoid distracting the dogs, (3) deaf-blind students without understandable speech could not give the dogs the necessary commands, and (4) deaf-blind travelers would not be appropriate dog guide users because they need assistance for certain aspects of travel, such as street crossings. This resistance to adapting training methods to accommodate deaf-blind students rendered most dog guide schools inaccessible to them. These schools had not considered training the dogs to understand nonverbal commands or communicating with the students using an interpreter or alternative methods of communication. Even when a deaf-blind person was accepted, staff at some schools insisted that the instruction be given verbally, rather than by print on palm or another method.

Fortunately, many schools now accommodate the communication needs of deaf-blind applicants and are interested in learning how to do so. They also understand that there are many aspects of independent mobility, of which street crossing is only one. The deaf-blind person and his or her dog can be an effective team, traveling independently most of the time and seeking assistance when needed.

Guiding Eyes for the Blind was a pioneer in this field and has been accepting deaf-blind students since the mid 1960s. It has successfully trained deaf and hearing-impaired individuals, some of whom were totally blind and profoundly deaf, including one who does not have understandable speech. Many of these graduates are now working with their second or third dog guides.

When Guiding Eyes for the Blind accepts a person who is deaf-blind for training after an on-site interview and assessment, they choose a dog that can handle the added responsibilities and pressures of working with an individual who is both blind and deaf. The dog is then trained specifically for that applicant, based on the individual's situation, mobility skills, and type of travel planned.

When the dog is ready, the individual is scheduled for a class. If the dog is dropped from training after beginning to work with the student, the student goes home and returns when another suitable dog is ready. The training is provided one-on-one throughout, and the trainer immediately follows up the training in the person's community.

According to a survey of dog guide schools that I conducted in 1992 (reported in Appendix C), other schools have also accepted deaf students. Some of these students had not lost their hearing until after they were experienced dog guide users or had graduated from the schools. International Guiding Eyes graduated three students who were totally deaf when there was a trainer at their school who could sign. However, most schools accept applicants only if they are able to hear well enough to judge the flow of traffic or hear vehicular traffic and to understand the lectures. Several schools require the applicants to have understandable speech. To this date, Fidelco Guide Dog Foundation will not accept applicants who are deaf-blind because thus far it has had no experience with them, nor will Eye Dog Foundation because it believes that applicants must be able to hear to use dog guides properly.

Several respondents to the survey indicated their desire to learn more about deaf-blindness and communication methods so they could consider how to adapt their programs to deaf-blind students. One school stated that if the communication problem could be overcome (for example, with an interpreter), deaf-blind applicants would be accepted.

It is important that deaf-blind travelers who use dog guides understand their abilities and their limitations and know when they need assistance. They should learn these things while they are being trained at the dog guide school and during follow-ups in their home areas by the trainer. (For information on the feasibility of crossing streets independently, see "Dog Guides" in Chapter 8. For the philosophy of various dog guide schools on this issue, see Appendix C.)

CHAPTER 8

STREET CROSSINGS

Other than communication issues, the one aspect of O&M training that is significantly different for people who are deaf-blind is the crossing of streets. People first need to know how reliably and in what situations they can determine the appropriate time to cross. If they cannot make these determinations, they will have to decide which intersections (driveways, avenues, or streets) they feel safe crossing by themselves (or with their dog guide) and which they will need to avoid or cross only with assistance. They must know how to get that assistance effectively and be familiar with some alternatives when they cannot get help.

DETECTING VEHICLES

People who have limited vision and hearing need to know whether they can detect vehicles well enough to cross streets safely when they do not want to depend on drivers to slow down for them. Several people (including Dan Smith and Steve Rhinne, O&M specialists at the Veterans Administration Blind Rehabilitation Center in Hines, Illinois) have attempted to develop a device that can detect vehicles. A radar traffic detector was adapted to detect vehicles approaching up to a third of a mile away, but because of lack of funds and concern about possible health side effects of the device's radar, it has not been developed further.

Crossing Intersections with No Traffic Light

In my experience, many visually impaired people (both hearing and deaf), especially those who recently lost their vision or hearing, have an unrealistic perception of their ability to detect vehicles. A few people whose loss of vision or hearing was slight are terrified to cross even quiet residential streets. Others who have significant visual and hearing impairments think they can still notice traffic well enough to cross busy streets safely.

People can gain a more realistic understanding of their own safety by analyzing their detection of vehicles at various intersections. These analyses can be more productive if the client and I use the timing method for limited detection (TMLD) and the timing method for unlimited detection (TMUD) (see Sauerburger, 1989). These timing methods can not only help people learn how effectively they can detect vehicles under various conditions, but enable them to become more aware of the specific effect that various conditions (such as masking sounds, hills, speed of the traffic, and lighting conditions) have on their detection of vehicles.

People's ability to judge whether the conditions are suitable for a safe crossing can also be assessed and improved. They first observe the situation at a certain intersection and decide whether they think they can detect the vehicles well enough to cross, then they and the instructor use the TMLD or TMUD to test their judgment.

Deaf people who have limited vision may improve their ability to see approaching vehicles by learning to use their vision as efficiently as possible. For example, people with a loss of central vision may learn to view the traffic eccentrically. When deaf people with restricted visual fields watch for oncoming traffic, they may see that the road is clear at a distance but may miss a car that is approaching nearby because they glance quickly, not realizing that their remaining central vision is not effective for scanning in this manner. Thus they must develop a scanning technique that enables them to observe the entire street; such a technique usually involves moving their eyes more slowly than they are accustomed to doing. They may be able to learn the speed they need to scan if they practice moving their eyes at various speeds while reporting if they see oncoming cars; the instructor can inform them if they are missing any cars.

One scanning technique that has worked for some people is to first look to the right, then scan all the way to the left slowly enough to see any cars approaching. If the coast is clear, they start to cross while scanning again for more cars from the right (starting straight ahead and scanning to the right). If they observe a car coming, they either go back and begin the process again, or if they can judge that the car is slow enough or far enough away, they complete the crossing. The ability to judge the speed and distance of cars can be tested using the TMUD (Sauerburger, 1989).

Crossing Intersections with Traffic Lights

At intersections with traffic lights, deaf people with limited but functional vision often need to learn how to watch the traffic to determine its cycle so they can determine when is the best time to cross. As is often the case with hearing visually impaired people, many deaf visually impaired people are not aware that they can cross more safely by analyzing the traffic pattern.

The deaf visually impaired person can practice assessing increasingly complicated intersections to figure out the cycle and the right time to cross, in the same manner that hearing blind people do. Of course, clients should be aware that the cycle of many intersections, especially those with separate signals for left-turning vehicles, varies, depending on the amount of traffic. They should also know that the function of many pedestrian-walk buttons is to prolong the green light (especially at wide streets where the light is not usually green long enough to allow a person to cross).

As they cross, these people should be aware of where they need to direct their limited vision to be alert to vehicles that are turning in front of them. If their vision has changed, they may not realize that they now need to modify the way they look for cars. For example, mobility instructor Mary Michaud-Cooney indicated that many deaf people with restricted visual fields failed to look behind and over their shoulders for turning traffic—something they did not have to do when they had full visual fields.

Travelers need to be alert to three possible sources of danger as they cross: vehicles turning left from the middle of the parallel street, vehicles turning right from the parallel street, and vehicles turning right on red from the perpendicular street. They should also know when they need to look in which direction. For example, a person who is starting to cross at a standard intersection with the parallel street on the left will need to first watch for vehicles turning from the parallel street (both from ahead and from behind). Once he or she reaches the middle of the street, there is no more concern from those sources. When approaching the last lane, the person should look to the right for possible right-turn-on-red vehicles.

At intersections with such variations as one-way streets, left-turning arrows, or islands separating the lanes where traffic turns right, the traveler may not need to watch for all three dangers for each crossing. With practice, he or she should be able to make this determination confidently and independently at new intersections and plan the safest way to cross.

Deaf visually impaired travelers who cross by following pedestrians should be skilled in how to do so. They should not cross just because two or three people start to cross, since those people may be going against the light and dodging the cars. Also, they should not cross with other people unless they are already aware that the part of the traffic cycle during which they want to cross is about to begin. They can then use the surge of a crowd to confirm that it is time to cross and to help shield them against turning cars.

The crowd may slow down to let a car cut in front, or it may be crossing during a break in traffic, rather than at a green light. Thus, visually impaired travelers who are relying on the crowd should cross *with* it, rather than walk ahead of or behind the people. Deaf travelers who use visual clues may find this difficult to do because they may be tempted to follow the crowd from behind, where they can see it more easily, or may continue ahead of the crowd without realizing it has stopped for a car. One person was convinced of the danger of using a crowd improperly when the crowd she was following stepped off the median strip just when the light was changing to red. Because she started to cross after they had started, rather than with them, the light had already changed to red when she stepped out. A car speeding toward the intersection from her right would probably have hit her if she had not been pulled back. If the person cannot independently know when it is time to cross and cannot use crowds properly, it would be best for him or her to ask for assistance and cross using a pedestrian as a guide.

WHEN VEHICLES CANNOT BE DETECTED

The rest of this chapter deals with issues and suggestions for situations in which people cannot hear or see well enough to detect vehicles. In such circumstances, the person must choose to cross only with assistance, avoid the intersection, or risk crossing alone. When they decide to cross alone, they are dependent on drivers to see them and avoid hitting them, since they cannot see or hear the vehicles well enough.

Is such a crossing safe? To answer this question, one must consider what is meant by the word *safe*. Lowrance (1976, quoted in Kraft, 1988, p. 189) concluded that "a thing is safe if its risks are judged to be acceptable." That is, each person has to decide whether the risk of such a crossing is acceptable. What one person considers "safe," another person will consider "unsafe."

Decisions About Crossing Without Assistance

Independent travelers need to consider crossing a wide range of intersections, including neighbors' driveways, entrances to parking lots and shopping centers, campus lanes, alleys, short dead-end streets, residential streets with stop signs, quiet streets with no stop signs, urban intersections, and highways. There is an element of danger at all of these intersections. Periodically, we hear about children being accidentally run over and killed by family members in their own driveways. Yet most travelers who are totally blind and profoundly deaf consider the danger of crossing their neighbors' driveways to be negligible and certainly worth the risk of crossing alone. However, most travelers who are deaf-blind consider the risk of crossing a busy urban street without assistance to be too great.

Each deaf-blind person must decide in which situations the risks are too great to cross alone. This decision must be based on objective information about the situation: how much risk there is, how feasible it is to get assistance, how much effort or expense is involved in planning alternative routes or using other transportation, and so forth. Nevertheless, the decision to cross at a certain place is subjective, as are all decisions. It is determined by peoples' judgment about how much risk is worth taking, how badly they want to get to their destination, and the value they place on the expense or effort or loss of autonomy involved in alternative plans.

The instructor's role is to help the deaf-blind person gather the objective data needed to make a decision. The decision, however, is the client's. At isolated neighborhood streets where there is only occasional traffic and at relatively quiet intersections where the vehicles must pull up to a stop sign, some people consider the danger small enough to risk crossing alone. Other people do not want to accept that risk, no matter how small it is.

When clients ask me what I suggest, I can only tell them what I would do in that situation if I had their skills. I try to make it clear that my decision is based on my own values—such as how much risk I am willing to take, how badly I would want to get to the destination, whether I would mind waiting half an hour for assistance or walking a few extra blocks to avoid the intersection, how much I trust drivers, whether I would prefer to pay for paratransit or alternative choices, and how I would feel about asking a friend for a ride. Different instructors would probably make different recommendations. The deaf-blind person must weigh his or her own values to come up with his or her own decision.

People who cannot see or hear the vehicles will need assistance to gather the objective information needed to make these decisions for each driveway or street. The instructor or a friend can stand with the person at various times during the day and describe what is happening, so he or she will know how frequently vehicles and people pass at that time of day. By pointing to the vehicles as they go by, you can indicate how fast they are going. Sometimes clients and I set up a signal system so they can learn about the traffic on a new street as they walk along it. I may move my finger across their shoulders or up and down their back to represent passing vehicles and to indicate the direction of the movement and the relative speed of the vehicles. You should also describe how visible the person is to drivers who may cross his or her path. On the basis of all this information, the deaf-blind person will then decide whether to risk crossing a particular street alone.

If clients make what seem to be reckless decisions about crossings, it may be because they do not have all the information. Several times, I was approached by distressed friends or colleagues of deaf-blind people who made rash crossings while cars screeched to a halt right in front of them. Sometimes deaf-blind people cross rashly because they do not care about the risk. Sometimes, however, they are not aware of the danger in which they have placed themselves or the panic and distress they have caused drivers. One person did not realize that drivers at that intersection could not see him until they were nearly upon him. Another believed that carrying a white cane would part the waters and make his crossings safe because the drivers would stop for it. Make sure clients have all the information they need, including how drivers react to them and their cane.

People who are naive or developmentally disabled may need to learn the concept of being safe versus being in danger before they can travel near streets. The concept of danger and safety can be built upon the observation that some things can cause pain (hot appliances and liquids, sharp needles and pins, and so on) and are therefore dangerous unless they are treated with caution and proper safety techniques. They need to understand that the street can be a dangerous place and that it should be treated with caution and respect. Effective role modeling is helpful; they can observe that when their guide takes them across streets, he or she is alert and cautious before starting.

They should also learn that in dangerous places, they need to follow whatever safety procedures would be appropriate for them. That is, those who have enough hearing or vision must learn to listen or look before crossing. Others must learn never to step off the curb or go down the ramp without assistance or, if the intersection is safe enough to cross independently, to stop and warn drivers of their intention to cross. People who have limited experience also need to develop the necessary judgment to determine which situations are safe enough to cross alone and which pose a risk greater than they are willing to accept.

Drivers' Awareness of the Traveler

If the deaf-blind person decides that a driveway, alley, business entrance, or street is isolated enough to risk crossing independently, he or she may wish to increase the chances of safety by warning the occasional driver who may be passing. One way to do so is to stop at the edge or curb and hold the cane out ahead, then put it back down and start to cross. If parked cars may be blocking the view, the traveler can warn drivers while standing at the curb, then walk a few feet into the street where he or she could be seen in case there were parked cars, and stop to warn the drivers again. The traveler might also alert drivers in the area that a deaf-blind person will be crossing there, in such ways as requesting that signs reading "DEAF-BLIND PEDESTRIAN" be installed at crosswalks or by distributing flyers to or visiting nearby homes and other buildings.

The person who is deaf-blind should be aware, however, that many drivers do not realize the meaning of the white cane (or do not care). Even though this warning may be effective for most drivers on a quiet street, an occasional driver may not stop. (For example, even at a small road on the campus of the Maryland School for the Blind, some drivers did not stop for a student holding out a white cane and a small replica of a stop sign.) Therefore, make sure that the traveler knows that holding out the white cane will not necessarily stop traffic.

Apparently, drivers in various states and provinces have differing routines. In Quebec, Eric St. Pierre, general director of the dog guide school Foundation Mira (see Resources), reports that drivers reliably stop for white canes and dog guides. At intersections with no traffic light, deaf-blind graduates of the school hold out a small stop sign for five seconds before crossing with their dog guides, and the drivers stop for them dependably. The stop sign is normally used by school traffic guards and is obtained from the local police department after permission is granted to use it in appropriate circumstances.

I decided to try stopping traffic with a sign in several residential communities in Maryland. I made a sign that looked like an authentic stop sign, with large white letters saying "DEAF-BLIND" instead of "STOP." The sign was about 10 inches high, identical on both sides, and easy to see. I wore sunglasses and stood at the curb with a cane in one hand and the sign in the other. When I heard a vehicle coming, I held the sign out so it was visible to drivers coming from either way for about five seconds, then raised my cane forward, lowered it, and (regardless of whether the car stopped) started walking steadily across. I did so about six times each in two quiet residential areas.

In both areas, some drivers stopped or slowed down for me or went around me, although a few halted with brakes screeching. One elderly lady coming from the right actually honked and sped up, passing within inches of me as I walked. If I had walked just a little faster, she would probably have been unable to avoid hitting my cane or perhaps me.

I thought that perhaps the reason for the drivers' lack of cooperation was that they were not accustomed to seeing strangers in their own neighborhoods (particularly one who is deaf-blind). Therefore, Eleanor Macdonald (director of the Family Service Foundation's Institute on Deaf-Blindness in Lanham, Maryland) and I tried it again at a two-lane street in a business area. We chose this street not because we thought it might be a safe place for a person who is deaf-blind to cross, but because we wanted to see if drivers were more cooperative when asked to stop in an area where they would be less incredulous to see a "deaf-blind" pedestrian. In this area, all the drivers seemed to be aware of me, and each driver slowed down or stopped in plenty of time to avoid hitting me.

Thus, holding a sign out to warn drivers may be helpful for crossing entrances and quiet residential streets if the drivers are not incredulous to see a person who is deaf-blind in their community (as they may have been during my first experiments). Also, it may be that a standard traffic-guard sign as is used at Foundation Mira would be more effective than a custom-made one.

Travelers should be aware that if they are walking on the left side of a busy street, drivers coming out of driveways and side streets may not be watching for them. Several times, people who are deaf-blind, one of whom was using a dog guide, were hit in these situations, although no one was seriously hurt. One visually impaired hearing person was also bumped by a car that she did not expect to pull out as she walked in front of it. In each case, the driver was waiting to make a right turn into a busy street, watching the traffic to the left while moving forward, and thus was unaware that a pedestrian was coming from the right. Therefore, deaf-blind travelers may prefer to warn drivers or draw attention to themselves before they start to cross in these situations by standing at the edge of the driveway or entrance, tapping the cane loudly, and carefully raising it up and down once or blowing a whistle. At night, reflective clothing, a flashlight, or a lighted cane may increase the possibility of being seen.

Soliciting Aid to Cross Streets

Travelers who are deaf-blind can cross streets by soliciting aid from passersby, drivers, neighbors, and shopkeepers. Travelers usually get assistance by using a combination of gestures, a card or sign, their voice, a prerecorded message, or an attention-getting sound. Janice Adams, who is deaf-blind, asks for assistance verbally and reports that people respond more readily when she accompanies her request with gestures and body language. She leans forward or turns her head to the side, as if looking for someone to assist her. Other travelers hold up a card or sign or use a recorded message asking for assistance. The deaf-blind person should be familiar with several ways to solicit aid and choose those that are most comfortable and effective.

The person who is deaf-blind may also have to learn to be patient when using this method to cross streets. One deaf-blind man walked across a street alone during a red light after waiting for assistance just a few minutes because he assumed people were passing him by without helping when no one had come near.

When asking for assistance, people who cannot recognize when someone has approached them should let would-be helpers know they need to be contacted by touch. Otherwise, when people offer to help, they sometimes leave when the traveler does not respond.

While being guided across, it is important that the traveler take the guide's arm to remain in control (a review of the Hines break is helpful; see Glossary). Otherwise, some guides abandon the traveler halfway across, thinking that he or she will be safe, and others insist on continuing to guide once they reach the other side. After being taken across the street, some travelers have even allowed their guide to take them a block or two the wrong way when the guide mistakenly assumed that is where they wanted to go; this situation is more likely to occur when the person's communication is limited. Again, these problems can be avoided if the deaf-blind person has taken the guide's arm to be escorted across rather than let the guide take his or her arm. Once on the other side, the traveler should thank the guide, indicate that he or she is all right, and continue confidently on his or her way.

Soliciting Aid from Pedestrians

Much of the information in this section was compiled in 1991 by interviewing 71 people who passed by or helped deaf-blind people who were soliciting aid with a card (see Sauerburger and Jones, 1992). On the basis of the survey we found that to be effective in soliciting aid to cross a street, a deaf-blind person should: (1) give every indication that he or she wants help to cross by requesting assistance with a card, voice, gestures, or a recording and (2) stand at the curb, facing the street to be crossed.

It is important that the person demonstrate that he or she needs assistance. When we interviewed people who helped our subjects cross the street, many told us that they would not have stopped to help if the person had not been holding up the card to ask for assistance, because they know that many blind people do not need or do not like to be offered help. Several even said that they assume that any person who carries a white cane can cross streets independently.

The person should stand at the curb and face the street. We found that when the deaf-blind person held the card while standing near the corner but not at the curb, some passersby reported that it never occurred to them that the card was requesting assistance to cross; many never bothered to read it, and some even seemed to avoid passing near it. This phenomenon may help explain the strange results of an experiment by Florence and LaGrow (1989), who asked a deaf-blind woman to solicit aid to cross a street from 60 people by handing them a card that requested assistance, rather than by standing at the curb and holding up the card; only 4 of the 60 people helped.

When the traveler is not facing the street, the helper sometimes needs to ask which street he or she wants to cross. When the traveler does not respond, some helpers leave because they do not know what to do. To avoid this problem, one traveler who is deaf-blind routinely points to the street he wants to cross as soon as someone taps him.

Soliciting Aid from Drivers

Travelers who are deaf-blind sometimes need to cross intersections where there are few or no pedestrians from whom to solicit aid. I found that if the drivers recognize the traveler's need and if they can safely pull over, many are willing to get out and guide the deaf-blind traveler. Some drivers who pass the traveler even turn around and park at a convenient place to get out to help. One deaf-blind person uses this method at a busy intersection where a traffic light stops the drivers long enough to read his message. He usually only has to wait three or four minutes before a driver offers him assistance.

To inform the drivers of the need for assistance, the traveler can hold up a laminated sign that unfolds to about 8½ by 11 inches. To make our sign, we followed the principles involved in making cards. The words "Cross Street" were large enough to be seen from across the street. Immediately below them are the words "Tap Me" in large letters, followed by text and the enlarged words "Deaf and Blind." The traveler should hold the sign to be visible to drivers who may be waiting at a light or stop sign or who may be able to turn into a quiet street where they can leave their car briefly.

Electronic Devices

Vibrotactile Devices

A vibrotactile device can detect the sound of vehicles, but not well enough to indicate if it is safe to cross a street. One such device, TACTAID II+ or 7 (see Resources), transforms most sounds into frequencies with vibrations that can be felt with receptors placed on the wrist or chest. The device was designed to assist sighted deaf people with lipreading, but since I was aware of a deaf-blind traveler who uses it to cross streets, I tested an earlier version of the device, the TACTAID II, to see how effectively it can detect vehicles. At the various streets where the testing was conducted, the device did not detect approaching cars until they were too close (Sauerburger, 1987). Thus, such a device would generally not be useful for the deaf-blind traveler to confirm when he or she could safely cross streets. At entrances or quiet intersections where he or she has decided to risk crossing alone and depends on drivers to stop, however, the vibrotactile device may help him or her avoid walking into moving cars or stepping in front of them.

Vibrating and Audible Traffic Signals

At intersections with a traffic light where the traveler cannot tell when the light is green but can avoid turning vehicles and can cross without veering into busy parallel traffic, an audible, tactile traffic signal may be the solution (see Resources). Some people who are deaf-blind think they could cross safely if only they could tell when the light turns green. Be sure that they understand that drivers will assume that they can hear and avoid cars; even if they cross at a green light, drivers may cut them off and hit them. These vibratory traffic signals are best for travelers who can avoid turning cars.

One such traveler is a deaf-blind woman who uses a dog guide. She needs to cross a busy two-lane street at a traffic light. We decided that with the help of her dog guide, she would be able to avoid the turning vehicles and cross if she could determine when the light turned green. Therefore, we asked the traffic department to install a vibrating traffic signal box for her to feel at each side of the street; this is being pursued at the time of this writing. The traveler who cannot avoid turning cars can request that the traffic signal be altered so that pedestrians have a separate walk signal while the traffic waits.

Traffic Sensors

At many intersections, traffic signals are programmed to determine the sequence of lights based on whether there are any vehicles in certain lanes. To detect these vehicles, transportation departments install inductive loops under the pavement or radar detectors. Although it has not yet been tried, it would be possible to install these vehicle detectors for a deaf-blind traveler at an intersection with no traffic light.

For example, at a street where traffic is infrequent but hazardous, these traffic sensors could be installed in each direction to detect vehicles far enough from the intersection that the deaf-blind traveler has sufficient warning to make a safe crossing. The traffic sensors could be connected to output at the intersection in whatever form the traveler can use (auditory, tactile, or visual), to signal when a vehicle is approaching and has reached the inductive loops or entered the radar's range.

DOG GUIDES

Inexperienced people assume that a dog guide can enable deaf-blind travelers to cross streets independently. They believe that the dog guide initiates crossings for hearing-blind people or that the dog guide would keep a deaf-blind person from harm if he or she commanded the dog to cross at the wrong time.

This latter belief is only partly true. Hearing-blind people who use dog guides line up at the curb and wait until they judge that it is safe to cross and then give the dog the command, "Forward." If the person misjudges and gives the command when a car is approaching, the dog guide is trained to refuse the command ("intelligent disobedience") or avoid the vehicle while crossing. Therefore, people conclude that the deaf-blind person who cannot recognize when it is safe to cross could give the forward command every minute or so and rely on the dog to cross while dodging the traffic or to refuse to obey the commands until it is safe to cross. However, representatives of dog guide schools in the past have emphasized that it is not safe for a dog guide to be responsible for any such crossing.

Nevertheless, several dog guide users who cannot hear the traffic well enough to cross by themselves have used their dog guides to initiate crossings, and one hired a dog trainer to help teach the dog to do so. In 1992, I surveyed dog guide schools about their position on this issue (see Appendix C). Although some maintained that under no circumstances can a dog guide be responsible for such crossings, several representatives responded that a dog could handle this responsibility if it had the temperament and training to be able to do so and if the intersection was such that the dog could decide when it was unsafe to cross. However, they said that most traffic situations are too difficult for any dog to recognize when it is not safe to cross. Several respondents stated that the dog guide users must use experience and common sense to determine whether they can depend on their dogs to be responsible for a particular crossing.

Even when a dog can be responsible for certain crossings, its ability to avoid danger should not be used indiscriminantly. According to Doug Roberts of the Seeing Eye, if a dog is expected to do a high percentage of these "traffic checks," the extra stress and responsibility can result in the dog's "nervousness, loss of confidence, refusal to work, tension-related illness (colitis), and ineffective guidance." Ted Zubrycki of Guiding Eyes for the Blind noted that "constant forward commands into traffic [are] unsafe. . .and intelligent disobedience quickly turns into a refusal to cross streets if pressured by the user [to] try to outmaneuver traffic. What most people fail to understand is that the word *safe* is not in a dog's memory bank." Also, I have found that the tendency of some dog guide users to relax and assume that the dog will always be alert to hazards is dangerous and may have been the cause of several tragic mishaps of hearing blind people.

Thus, dog guides who can handle this task should not routinely be given the responsibility for crossing streets except in situations where the percentage of occurrences when the traveler commands the dog to cross at the wrong time is relatively low, such as at quiet, residential streets or when the traveler can hear or see well enough to detect most vehicles. To make such a crossing, according to Bradly Scott of Leader Dogs for the Blind, the traveler would line up and give the forward signal, then step off the curb and walk slowly for the first three or four steps before resuming his or her normal speed. This slow start helps drivers anticipate the traveler's direction of travel and gives the dog a greater opportunity to concentrate on approaching vehicles and to straighten the line of travel.

Any dog that is used for this purpose must be carefully chosen and trained. Keith Laber of Guide Dogs of the Desert stated that a dog that is expected to guide deaf-blind people across streets independently must have a certain sensitivity level, be bold enough to negotiate traffic, and yet demonstrate a respect for traffic.

Most of the dog guide schools that stated that dogs should never be responsible for street crossings will not accept deaf-blind students. The Eye Dog Foundation, for example, believes that hearing is required to use a dog guide properly. International Guiding Eyes requires deaf-blind graduates to sign a statement agreeing not to use the dog for independent crossings but to obtain assistance for all crossings, including on quiet residential streets. (For more information about dog guides for people who are deaf-blind, see "Deaf-Blind People and Dog Guides" in Chapter 7).

WHEN THERE IS NO WAY TO CROSS A STREET

Some routes are unrealistic for travelers who are deaf-blind because they involve crossings that would be too risky to cross independently and no assistance is available. In such circumstances, deaf-blind people might plan alternate routes; arrange for assistance from neighbors or shopkeepers; ride a bus to the end of the line and back to get on and off on their side of the street; or use taxis, carpools, or paratransit systems to avoid such situations.

In terms of mobility, the best place for independent travelers who are deaf-blind to live or work would be an area with many pedestrians (so assistance is available to cross streets) or one in which they can travel to and from a bus stop and other destinations without having to cross streets they think are too dangerous. If deaf-blind people are unable to use their mobility skills because they live where they cannot cross the streets or get assistance, the instructor may think that the training was a waste of time. Most mobility instructors have experienced similar problems with hearing-blind clients; after they learn how to travel independently, some hearing-blind clients rue the fact that they live where there is no public transportation and must continue to rely on other people to give them rides. Likewise, some deaf-blind clients with newly acquired skills regret that they live where they cannot walk farther than the corner. This situation does not necessarily mean that the mobility training was worthless. Once people realize their potential for independence, whether they are hearing or deaf, they may plan to move to an area where they can take advantage of their new abilities.

CHAPTER 9

TEACHING ORIENTATION AND MOBILITY TO PEOPLE WITH LIMITED LANGUAGE SKILLS

This chapter was written for O&M specialists who are already knowledgeable about assessing and teaching O&M to visually impaired and blind people, including those who are developmentally disabled. It presents a brief introduction to working with this underserved population—deaf-blind people whose communication or language skills are limited.

More information on working with this population can be found in publications about adults and children who are developmentally disabled, visually impaired, hearing impaired, or have multiple disabilities (see, for example, Chen & Smith, 1992; CNIB, 1992; *Community-Based Living Options*, 1987; Gee, Harrell, & Rosenberg, 1987; Geruschat, 1980; Goetz & Guess, 1987; Joffee, 1991; Signorat & Watson, 1981; *Strategies for Serving Deaf-Blind Clients*, 1984). The American Foundation for the Blind is compiling comprehensive teaching materials and resources for those who work with deaf-blind children, much of which will also be helpful to those who work with adults with limited language skills (for information, contact the American Foundation for the Blind; see Resources).

When working with deaf-blind adults who have limited language or communication skills, it is easy to underestimate or overestimate their abilities. Avoid making assumptions about their potential for understanding language, since some people lack language skills because they were not adequately exposed to language.

Program planning and instruction for these people is usually done by a team that includes professionals from various disciplines and family members. Among other things, the O&M instructor needs to ascertain the most useful techniques and routes for the client to learn and the best approach for communicating with and instructing him or her.

To do so, the instructor has to talk with those who spend time with the deaf-blind person and who know him or her best. The other service providers and the family members need to learn how to use and reinforce the O&M skills because most of the time, the deaf-blind person will be with them, not with the O&M instructor.

Some deaf-blind people with limited language are flexible about understanding several different signs for the same thing, and this is to be encouraged. If the person's capacity for communication is *very* limited, however, it is best for everyone to agree on and be consistent about the communication system that they use. Arlyce Watson, day program specialist at Family Service Foundation's Institute on Deaf-Blindness, suggested that it may help to record this communication system or the signs and symbols that the person can recognize, so new staff members and others can familiarize themselves with it.

COMMUNICATION SKILLS

People have limited language skills for many reasons. Some may have never been exposed sufficiently to any language system. For example, one woman with whom I worked seemed to have normal intelligence but had been institutionalized with mentally retarded people from the time she became deaf and blind at age 3 until she was about age 40. Therefore, she had few opportunities to learn any communication system. When I met her at age 50, she used gestures only.

Other people may have cognitive impairments as well as visual and hearing impairments. Many were also raised and taught by people who knew little or no sign language. You can imagine how much communication any person, especially if cognitively impaired, would learn if placed in an environment where people positioned or manipulated him or her without speaking a word except "eat," "stand up," and "bathroom." Yet I saw people who had visual and hearing impairments in schools and institutions with staff whose only interaction with them was gestures and the three or four signs the staff knew.

Communication is sometimes taught to children who are deaf-blind by using "object cues" to symbolize real objects. The object cue can be a real object (a piece of cereal to represent breakfast, glass to represent a drink, a key to represent a ride in the car) or part of a real object (a shoelace to represent shoes, a piece of coat fabric to signify it is time to get the coat and go outside). After the child grasps the meaning of such concrete object cues, these cues can be paired with increasingly abstract cues or symbols that can then be substituted for the more concrete symbold. Eventually standard signs are paired with the symbols so the child can understand their meaning.

However, sometimes when youngsters learn concrete symbols or made-up signs, they are never taught more abstract symbols or standard signs for those concepts. Well-meaning staff who do not know standard signs may teach them to understand such symbols as a tap on the shoulder to indicate "sit down" or two taps on the elbow to mean "time to eat." One deaf-blind person who came to the program where

I worked arrived with his own dictionary of signs that he understood and that had been made up by the staff at his last program. The staff at our program are deaf and used sign language with him. To make him feel at home in his new environment, they used his signs for a while, but paired the standard signs with his home signs. Before long, he understood the standard signs for all the items in his dictionary and had learned many more. People who have the capacity to learn made-up signs and symbols can just as easily learn standard signs, which allows them to communicate with others.

Although some instructors teach signs by manipulating the deaf-blind person's hands to form the signs, the deaf-blind person should eventually be able to recognize these signs using interactive tactile signing—the customary communication mode for deaf-blind people. With interactive tactile signing, the deaf-blind person places his or her hand or hands on those of the person who is signing. It is an efficient way for them to communicate; most signs can be perceived accurately in this manner without the signer's having to slow down. Deaf-blind people who use sign language have no difficulty tactilely learning new signs and do not need residual vision to recognize them.

Until recently, however, these facts were not commonly known among professionals who work with deaf-blind children or with adults whose primary language is English (rather than ASL). For example, Dinsmore (1959, p. 27) explained that to use signs, "the speaker takes the deaf-blind person's hands in his and moves them for him, forming the various signs wanted. As an alternative method, the deaf-blind person can place his hands on those of the speaker and follow his movements in making the signs, but this is somewhat more difficult. It would be almost impossible and certainly cumbersome to attempt to teach many signs to a blind person." Today, some staff and family members who are not familiar with interactive tactile sign language continue to manipulate the deaf-blind person's hands to make the signs. This method is inappropriate and more time consuming and cumbersome than is interactive tactile sign language.

Deaf-blind people who had limited opportunity to develop language skills as children can still improve their ability to communicate as adults if they are in a responsive environment filled with communication and interaction. Most of the residents of the group homes of Family Service Foundation's Institute on Deaf-Blindness in Lanham, Maryland, were adults when they arrived. They are deaf, legally or totally blind, and developmentally disabled. All the staff at these homes are fluent in sign language, and most of them are deaf. The residents are thus exposed to a lot of signs and nonverbal communication, and most of them have greatly improved their ability to understand others and to express themselves. One teacher who did not know sign language and who had worked with a resident before he came to this home visited him after he had lived there several years. She was surprised at the extent to which he could understand others and express himself.

Therefore, do not assume that your clients have reached their full potential for understanding language and expressing themselves. Whether the clients seem to understand or not, always explain what you are doing or what you expect (using the communication system the team has agreed upon, such as voice and signs, pictorial description, gestures, or object cues). Often, with enough exposure to language and communication, the client will learn the significance of phrases or words and respond accordingly (for example, "<time> <go> <home> <now>; <get> <your> <coat>").

However, do not overestimate how much clients can understand. If they do not respond appropriately, you must determine if it is because they do not understand the language (or signs or symbols) or the concept involved or if they understand both but cannot or will not perform the task. As with any client, the instructor and team members must use creative strategies to find out how much the deaf-blind person is able to understand and the best ways to teach him or her.

ASL (see "Communication with Sign Language" in Chapter 1) and pictorial descriptions (see "'Pictorial Description'" in Chapter 2) are often more effective with people with limited language than are signs used in English order. For example, one morning a young man who had been living in Family Service Foundation's program for a few months came to breakfast with his shoes on the wrong feet. His service provider, who is deaf and fluent in ASL, went to him and pointed to the shoes, made her hands into fists facing down (the sign for shoes, though he did not know it), then reversed her arms and pointed to the shoes again. He understood, and put his shoes on the correct feet. He would probably not have understood the signed English statement "<your> <shoes> <are> <on> <the> <wrong> <feet>; <take> <them> <off> <and> <put> <your> <shoes> <on> <the> <right> <feet>."

All of us feel less stressed if we know what to expect. "[N]ever act on a person with sensory impairments without first giving him/her information about what is about to happen" (Rowland & Stremel-Campbell, 1987, p. 65). It can be difficult to enable the deaf-blind person who has minimal communication skills to anticipate what will happen, but be creative and work with the team to develop ways of letting him or her know what to expect. If signs or symbols or objects are regularly used as cues for such things as work activities, a trip in the van, or time for meals or bedtime, the deaf-blind person may learn to recognize them and anticipate the trip or activity. Also, activities can be more easily anticipated if they are structured and scheduled consistently from day to day. If you wear a favorite cologne or aftershave lotion, your client may be able to use your scent to recognize or anticipate your presence (but do not overwhelm him or her with aromas).

ASSESSING VISION AND HEARING

The remaining vision and hearing of people who are deaf-blind and developmentally disabled can be assessed in the same way as for any person who is blind and developmentally disabled. Carefully observe cues, such as what the person reacts to, reaches for, or bumps into; how the lighting affects that ability; what sounds the person responds to; and whether the person can find the source of the sound. CNIB (1992) developed a functional curriculum for assessing the vision and hearing of deaf-blind adults, as well as their communication and O&M skills (see Canadian National Institute for the Blind in Resources).

The size of the client's visual field may be determined if one person gets the client's attention while the other person slowly brings an easily seen favorite item from the side toward the center of vision. When the client turns to look, it usually indicates that the item has entered his or her field of vision. Repeat this procedure on different occasions to be sure that the client's response was not a coincidence. One cooperative client would copy my hand shapes when he could see them both, changing shapes as I did. I then put one hand in front of my face, bringing my other hand so far to the side that I knew he could not see it. As I slowly moved the side hand toward my face, I changed the shapes of both hands. He watched the hand near my face and copied it until suddenly he turned his eyes and copied the other, indicating to me that my other hand had entered his field of vision.

If the client responds slowly, it may be difficult to know when he or she first sees the item. If the client can keep his or her gaze steadily on the first target, bring the second target toward the center in increments and hold it long enough to let the client react before bringing it closer to the center.

TEACHING O&M

Much that is true about teaching O&M to people who are visually impaired and developmentally disabled is also true about teaching those who are deaf as well. Many will need to learn the concept of safety and danger (see "Decisions About Crossing Without Assistance" in Chapter 8), as well as problem-solving and decision-making skills. They will usually require many trips before they learn a route. Most are more comfortable and learn best when they can follow well-established routines.

For a person to learn to travel independently, he or she must understand that there is an objective and want to reach the destination. Before starting each route, use appropriate signs, signals, words, or object cues to explain the purpose of the trip, so that eventually the client will understand what the destination is and be motivated to reach it.

Many O&M techniques and strategies that are effective for teaching people who are developmentally disabled and blind are just as effective with those who are also deaf. To help with orientation, a chair, table, or bedroom door can be identified with a symbol attached to it; for example, scissors can be placed on the jam of the craft door or a spoon on the jam of the cafeteria door. When starting the route, the deaf-blind person can be given a scissors or spoon and told that he or she is going to that destination (each place, as well as each person, should have a name-sign or symbol). For example, hand him or her a spoon and sign "<now> <time> <go-to> <cafeteria>" (using the name-sign for "cafeteria").

Once the client understands the meaning of the object cues, the cues can be arranged in a "calendar box," as is sometimes done with developmentally disabled people who are hearing and sighted. The box may consist of a row of bins, each with its own hinged lid, with the object cues in the bins in the order that the person will use them. For example, the first bin may contain scissors for the morning craft lesson; the second bin, a spoon for lunch; the third bin, bolts for industrial shop; and so on. The client can learn to follow the schedule throughout the day by checking to see what is in the next bin in the calendar box. Some people leave the lid open, bring the object cue to the activity, and return it to the open bin of the calendar box when the project or period is finished. This procedure can make transition to the next activity easier as they close the lid and search the next bin for the next object cue. Rustie Rothstein, a consultant on deaf-blindness, suggested that the objects can be carried easily in waist packs.

Usually it is important to teach people while they are doing meaningful tasks (Joffee, 1991; Lolli, 1980). They often do not understand the concept of practice, and will be frustrated if they are asked to go to the cafeteria when it is not time to eat or to practice walking outside with no destination that is meaningful to them. Some behavioral problems are a result of people not understanding that they are "practicing." Mobility instructors at the Helen Keller National Center for Deaf-Blind Youths and Adults have worked unusual hours because they needed to be on hand for "mobility lessons" when the clients wake up, find the shower and return, go to the cafeteria and eat, and head for their first class.

Thus, mobility instructors who work as consultants or as itinerant instructors have to provide thorough in-service training and work closely with the staff or family members so that techniques and routes can be taught consistently at the appropriate times. Because the staff or family members are usually with the person when the skills should be applied, it is they who will reinforce and teach the techniques introduced by the mobility instructor. The mobility instructor monitors the client's progress.

Sometimes I am able to have clients practice by walking with them to the destination and leaving something valuable there. For example, we may walk to the bathroom and together leave a toy, stuffed animal, or piece of candy on the sink. After we return to where we started, I sign or say, "Where's the [toy/animal/candy]? Let's get the [toy/animal/candy]!" We work our way back to the bathroom while I teach or reinforce skills and then return. If the client is well oriented and understands me, he or she will retrieve the item alone while I observe and evaluate. Some clients will agree to run errands while the instructor teaches and reinforces skills and routes ("<Please> <go-to> <Jones> <office>. <Paper> <give-to> <Jones> <please>"). Outside, I have occasionally hidden "treasures" that clients can try to find near landmarks that I want them to find and identify, such as fire hydrants and bus stop signs.

With people with developmental disabilities, the majority of teaching usually involves physical demonstrations (with the client observing visually or tactilely) and positioning and manipulating the client to use the technique being taught (Joffee, 1991; Lolli, 1980; Primrose-McGowan, 1980). Cane techniques and positions for trailing or protecting oneself can be taught hand over hand as the client walks.

The ideal routes in which to practice these skills are those that the deaf-blind person may be motivated to learn, that require skills that can be used regularly, and that he or she normally travels at a time when staff or family members have the time to teach or reinforce them. The route should be broken down into manageable segments to learn (Gee, Harrell, & Rosenberg, 1987). All techniques and concepts should be taught using appropriate communication, so the client can learn the signs or symbols associated with them. For example, on several lessons when guiding one client, I signed "right" or "left" every time I turned. She learned to turn the correct way if I signed "left" or "right" as she walked.

COMMUNITY AWARENESS*

When working with deaf-blind people with limited language, one of the most important things to keep in mind is their need for awareness of the community. They can be involved in such activities as shopping, banking, using the laundromat and post office, going to the shoe repair shop, fast-food restaurants, and recreational activities. Often, they have not been given opportunities to do so because they were not completely independent or because, with their lack of communication skills or inappropriate behavior, it was easier for the family or group home staff to take care of their shopping or personal needs without involving them.

Yet it is essential for staff and families to allow people who are deaf-blind to participate in community activities in whatever way they can, even if they are only able to do part of the activities themselves. Many of these individuals will never be totally independent in the community, but that should not stop O&M instructors from teaching them to do what they can. The more opportunities they have to learn and to grow, the more they can understand about their world and the choices available to them. With this approach, it is more likely that they will achieve their potential for independence.

COMMUNICATING WITH THE PUBLIC

The instructor and team members can be creative in developing ways for people with limited language to communicate with the public well enough to accomplish what

*This section was written by Mary Michaud-Cooney, O&M specialist and deaf-blind consultant.

they need (see also Chapter 3). Some people bring empty containers of desired products to the store to help them match and find the products (if they have enough vision) or to help explain to the salespeople what they want. The "communication book" is also effective. The communication book is a notebook, paper, poster, or set of cards designed with symbols of concepts and objects (such as pictures of a milkshake, toilet, or hairbrush). The client who learns what the symbols mean can point to them to request things or to express feelings.

Items in the communication book can be pictures (drawn or cut from advertisements or labels), textured squares and tactile symbols, printed words, or anything that the client can learn to recognize. A simple communication book may have a paper plate glued to a page for the deaf-blind person to indicate that he or she is hungry and a paper cup to indicate the desire for a drink. For people who have enough vision, some communication books (or materials to make one) are available through catalogues (see Resources).

Communication books for independent or semiindependent travelers could have pictures or tactile graphics accompanied by the printed words or messages to indicate to the public what the deaf-blind person wants. The instructor and client or team can be creative when designing the book to suit the client's needs and come up with symbols that the client can learn to identify. For example, the deaf-blind person could bring his or her book to the counter of a favorite fast-food restaurant and point to the pictures or tactile symbols for "burger and fries." Cards can also be made or purchased with pictures of items needed from the store to bring as a "shopping list."

The response of the public can be understood by the person with limited language skills if it is structured so he or she will understand it (see "Public Responses" in Chapter 3). The creative instructor can work with the client to come up with whatever structured response he or she will understand in that situation.

TEACHING THE CLIENT TO HANDLE AN EMERGENCY

Because there can never be certainty that things will go as planned, no person can be a fully independent traveler unless he or she knows what to do when plans do not go as expected. For example, a hearing-sighted man who is mentally retarded was taught how to take the bus to work. After three years of commuting without incident, he accidentally boarded the bus that goes downtown. He did not know how to take the bus back or telephone home for help, so he lived on the streets until he was found three days later. Only then was he taught how to find and use a telephone for assistance.

People with limited language ability who can travel independently must also learn how to handle unexpected situations. They should carry identification and emergency telephone numbers and know what to do with them, or they should

> **I AM LOST OR NEED HELP.** My name is __________ and I am deaf and can't see well. Please call one of these numbers and tell them where I am.
>
> **Thank you!**
>
> (202) ___-_________ (home)
>
> (202) ___-_________ ("Deaf Aid Program")
>
> (If no one answers these numbers, please call the police, and tell them I am lost or need assistance).

Figure 1. Card for use in an emergency.

carry a card that explains that they need someone to help them call certain telephone numbers for assistance (see Figure 1). Making sure that the deaf-blind person understands how to use this card can be tricky and time consuming, but it is necessary.

After one young man who is developmentally disabled and has Usher's syndrome had learned to travel to and from his day program by bus, he was given the card pictured here. To learn how to use it, he was "stranded" several times with me or with a staff person from his day program. The staff person and I took turns serving as role models to teach him to find a stranger or salesperson to whom he could give the card and a quarter to make the phone call. On his trial run he went into a store and gave the card to a salesperson, who made the phone call for him. However, he then left before anyone could have come for him. We repeated the experience in a variety of places in which one of us was with or near him. The other person would leave us both "stranded" and return to the agency to wait by the phone. After about seven trials, the client finally understood what to do. After the other staff person dropped us off and we did a little shopping, I signed that we needed to get home, but "<our> <ride> <GONE!> <What to do!> <What to do!>" He went by himself to a store, reached into his pocket for the card and the emergency quarter, gave them to a salesperson, and waited alone in the store about 20 minutes until help arrived. He now takes the bus to and from his day program by himself, and we can sleep nights knowing that he understands what to do if he is lost or stranded!

It is also important for people to be able to reach safety during an emergency at home. At the Helen Keller National Center for Deaf-Blind Youths and Adults, mobility instructor Doug McJannet and behavioral specialist John Walters trained people who are developmentally disabled and deaf-blind what to do when an alarm goes off in their dormitory. Their practical approach is described in detail in *Community-Based Living Options for Young Adults with Deaf-Blindness* (1987).

APPENDIX A

INSTRUCTIONS FOR MAKING A MOBILITY MUFF

A "mobility muff" is a muff for two people to use to keep their hands warm while using tactile communication. These instructions describe how to make a lined muff with a cuff on each end. However, you can sew, knit, or even buy a muff of any size, lined or unlined, with elastic or velcro instead of cuffs, or whatever you like, as long as it is big enough for two people to move their hands around inside. This muff is just big enough for me to fingerspell comfortably into someone else's hand, but if you have large hands or want more movement for signs, make it big enough for you to move around inside it.

MATERIALS

Two pieces of stretch fabric, such as stretch velour, each 14 inches by 18 inches wide (one is for the muff and one is for the lining). The direction of the stretch should be along the 18-inch ends. You can make the muff from fabric that does not stretch if you make it larger.

Two pieces of ribbed material, each 5 inches by 6 inches (for the cuffs). The direction of the stretch is along the 6-inch end. The width may need to vary from 6 inches, depending on how much the ribbing stretches; make it wide enough to stretch around someone's coat sleeve and add enough for the seam allowance.

INSTRUCTIONS

1. For each of the four pieces, sew the sides together to make four separate tubes; press the seams. The tubes that are the muff and lining will each be 14 inches long and about 8¾ inches wide when flat; the tubes that will make the cuffs will each be 5 inches long and about 2¾ inches wide.
2. To make the muff, turn one muff tube inside out (so the seam edges are inside the tube). Put the other muff tube inside the first (the seam edges should be sandwiched between the tubes). You now have a lined muff.
3. To make the cuffs, take one end of each cuff tube and double it over until you have the two ends together (seam edges should be hidden inside the cuff).
4. With the edges together, pin one cuff evenly around the outside of one end of the muff (you will have to stretch the cuff a *lot*). Sew the edge of the cuff to the edge of the muff and turn the cuff right side out. Press the seam. Do the same for the other cuff.
5. You should now have a muff with a cuff on each end.

APPENDIX B

EXPERIMENTS IN SENSORY DEPRIVATION

During the 1950s and 1960s, experiments that were originally conducted to investigate the effects of brainwashing showed that normal people experience various cognitive and perceptual changes during sensory deprivation. These changes include enhanced or impaired thought processes, hallucinations, and susceptibility to suggestion and persuasion (see Mendelson et al., 1964; Slade & Bentall, 1988; Solomon et al., 1965; Zubek, 1969).

It is not clear whether the information about sensory deprivation derived from these experiments applies to the experience of deaf-blind people. Many of the changes caused by the deprivation decreased as the subjects adapted to the condition. Whether the subjects experienced sensory deprivation in one long session or in several shorter sessions (in one case the sessions were a year apart), after about 24 accumulated hours of sensory deprivation, many of its effects began to decrease (Zubek, 1969, p. 146). One exception was the effect of hallucinations, which increased and became more formed and complex after 24 hours.

These experiments tested the effects of a wide range of sensory deprivation. Many subjects received homogeneous stimulation, such as white noise or repetitive sounds, or diffused light seen through opaque goggles or through the inside of a small dome. More complete sensory deprivation was achieved by having the subjects' vision occluded by darkness or eye patches and their hearing cut off with headphones or by being in a soundproof room. Some experimenters also inhibited their tactile sense (by putting mitts on their hands) and their kinesthetic sense (by strapping their arms or legs to prevent the joints from moving). Some subjects were placed in respirators (iron lungs) with a box built around the head, and others were submerged in a tank of water while wearing a special breathing mask (see Zubek, 1969, pp. 18–27).

Total sensory deprivation apparently is not necessary to experience the cognitive changes and hallucinations. In fact, compared to relatively complete sensory deprivation, the homogeneous sensory stimulation (opaque goggles and white noise) produced more cognitive and perceptual impairment, and both conditions seem equally conducive to inducing complex hallucinations. The sensory deprivation achieved in the water tank did not produce significantly more imaginary experiences than did other methods of sensory deprivation (Zubek, 1969, pp. 50–51, 115).

Sensory deprivation altered the intellectual performance of many subjects. During the experience, they found it difficult to concentrate, and their thought processes rapidly accelerated and moved quickly from one subject to another. Unstructured behaviors, such as speaking, generating ideas, and creating stories, were considerably impaired; moderately structured tasks, including problem solving, were somewhat impaired, and highly structured tasks, such as retention and learning, were either unaffected or facilitated.

In one study (Zubek, 1969), the subjects listened to a passage from *War and Peace* and answered questions to test their retention of the information. Half the subjects then underwent an hour of sensory deprivation, after which they were given another test that they hadn't expected. These subjects not only did better than those who had not undergone sensory deprivation, they did better than they had done immediately after hearing the passage—even though all but one subject reported that they had not thought about the passage during the sensory deprivation.

The effects of sensory deprivation disappeared after the experience. Subjects who had undergone two weeks of the deprivation returned to normal in an average of 3½ days (the longest time was 8 days).

In most cases, the subjects found the sensory deprivation experience unpleasant and stressful and often withdrew from the experiment before the designated time. Many of the effects (except hallucinations) could be decreased by purposeful exercise and were increased when the subject's movement was restricted. However, varying the amount of movement that the subject was permitted in the chamber seemed to have no effect (Zubek, 1969).

HALLUCINATIONS

Although some of the imagery the subjects experienced during the sensory deprivation was auditory or somasthetic, most of it was visual, similar to that caused by taking hallucinatory drugs. The phenomena varied enormously from person to person (Slade & Bentall, 1988, p. 15). Some hallucinations, called Type A, were simple perceived imagery, such as seeing flashes of light or geometric figures or hearing tones or clicks. Type B hallucinations were complex, integrated, formed hallucinations of landscapes or scenes of people, animals or cartoonlike characters, voices, and the like. Some subjects reported that these hallucinations were like having a dream while awake. Auditory hallucinations were perceived as if they were coming from outside the person (Slade & Bentall, 1988; Zubek, 1969).

The reports of hallucinations from early experiments were exaggerated because they did not differentiate between Type A and Type B hallucinations (Slade & Bentall, 1988; Solomon et al., 1965; Zubek, 1969). Later studies showed that about half the subjects experienced some kind of imagery, and only 5–20 percent had Type B hallucinations (Zubek, 1969). The longer that people experienced the sensory deprivation, the more complex was their imagery; those who had Type B hallucinations usually did so only after 24 hours of sensory deprivation (Slade & Bentall, 1988; Zubek, 1969).

Many of the subjects were at first amused by the hallucinations but later found them irritating and sometimes were kept awake by them. Most realized that the hallucinations were not real, but in one study 3 of the 27 people who perceived imagery thought that they were real. Subjects had a small degree of control over the hallucinations; they could see objects that were suggested by the experimenters, but not in the intended form (Zubek, 1969).

The hallucinations usually disappeared or decreased during complex mental activity, such as math problems, and sometimes during meaningful interaction with others. However, they did not disappear during exercise or conversation. In a study using sets of two male strangers in twin respirators, 20 percent hallucinated. When the subjects were a husband and a wife, they talked more, the conversation was more intimate, and only 5 percent hallucinated (Zubek, 1969).

One experiment studied the effects of sensory deprivation on 20 profoundly deaf students at Gallaudet College (Mendelson et al., 1964). Ten subjects sat quietly for an hour while looking at placid pictures on the wall, and a week later they sat in the same room for an hour wearing opaque goggles. The other 10 subjects did the same in reverse order. Most subjects experienced some imagery in both sessions. As with other subjects, their imagery was primarily visual, along with some somasthetic and a few auditory sensations. The subjects had more perceived imagery during the first session than during the second, which the authors speculated might be because of their higher anxiety. On average, however, the students experienced significantly more imagery when their vision was occluded with the goggles than when they could look at the pictures. The subjects reported that the imagery was unlike their usual daydreams or night dreams and but was a unique form of visual imagery for them.

This study is interesting not only because of its findings concerning the effect of deprivation of vision on deaf people, but because the authors mentioned that researchers at that time were apparently reluctant to work with deaf subjects because of the language barrier. Among other things, Mendelson's group set out to determine whether the "language of signs" would be adequate for communicating concepts and nuances of thought; they concluded that deaf subjects can be utilized when adequate provision is made for communication.

SUSCEPTIBILITY TO PERSUASION

Compared to control subjects under normal conditions, subjects undergoing sensory deprivation were found to be more susceptible to suggestion (Suedfeld, 1969). That is, they were more likely to perceive things the way the experimenter wanted them to. Sensory deprivation also rendered people with "simple" personalities more susceptible to persuasion. That is, their attitude or opinion was more easily changed if they heard the information or propaganda during sensory deprivation.

A *simple personality* was defined as one whose information processing is rigid and externally determined. They are less able to integrate new information into their conceptual structures without changing those structures or attitudes. A *complex personality* is one whose information processing is flexible, finely differentiated, and internally controlled and who can accept dissonance more easily. Such people are not more likely to change their attitudes during sensory deprivation than during normal conditions.

To receive stimulation as a reward, subjects undergoing sensory deprivation would comply more readily with the experimenters than would those under normal conditions. However, the stimulation that they craved was not just any stimulation or even varied stimulation; it was "informational stimulation," which was defined as sounds or events that were unpredictable. For example, the subjects were not motivated to cooperate to receive even complex stimulation if it was predictable (such as a complex repeated pattern), but they were motivated to receive random patterns and such otherwise boring stimuli as propaganda and stock prices if they were new. Even though they were more cooperative with the experimenters when they were experiencing sensory deprivation, those who recognized the intent of the propaganda rejected it more strongly when under sensory deprivation than when under normal conditions (Suedfeld, 1969; Zubek, 1969). Subjects who were deprived of only one sense, for example, sight, were not motivated to comply if they continued to receive highly valued information in another sense, such as hearing (Zubek, 1969).

According to Suedfeld (1969, p. 166), the subjects were more susceptible to suggestion and persuasion because of the "lack of informational anchors in the sensory deprivation situation. The subject is at loose ends, without guidelines for his behavior, unable to concentrate, and in a state of stimulus- and information-hunger. (He's completely in the dark, in other words.) This condition has the effect of maximizing the impact and the reward value of whatever information *is* available to him."

APPENDIX C

SURVEY OF DOG GUIDE SCHOOLS

School[a]	*Will the school accept deaf-blind or hard-of-hearing students? If so, are there any stipulations?*[b]	*Does the school agree that dog guides can share responsibility for certain street crossings? If so, under what conditions?*
Canadian Guide Dogs for the Blind	School does not accept deaf-blind students, though it does accept those with hearing loss if they can localize sounds and independently initiate safe street crossings.	No, the traveler should be responsible for all street crossings because "intelligent disobedience" should be relied on only as a last report, not as a strategy for routine street crossings.
Canine Vision Canada	Yes, the school has accepted blind people with hearing impairments and would accept a profoundly deaf-blind student. The school has trained some dogs whose primary function is guiding the traveler but who also have limited duties as a hearing dog in the home (being careful not to load the dog with too many responsibilities). The school also trains dogs for people who are deaf only or physically disabled.	Not certain; has had no experience with travelers who cannot hear or see the vehicles well enough to cross independently.
Eye Dog Foundation for the Blind	The school does not accept deaf-blind students, stating that the proper use of dog guides requires hearing.	No, the use of dog guides requires that dogs obey their masters, and for proper use, their masters should direct their dog guides where needed.
Eye of the Pacific Guide Dogs and Mobility Services	The school has no set policy; thus far it has had no deaf-blind applicants.	Did not respond.
Fidelco Guide Dog Foundation	The school does not accept deaf-blind students because it has had no experience working with people who are deaf-blind.	No, Fidelco guides are educated to be cautious in traffic, but the person has to make the primary judgment of traffic at each intersection. This primary responsibility cannot be delegated to the dog.

[a] The addresses of the schools appear in Resources. The survey was conducted in 1992.

[b] Some schools emphasized that deaf-blind students would have to meet the criteria required of any student, such as prerequisite orientation and mobility skills.

Foundation Mira	Yes, for 10 years the school has graduated blind people who are profoundly deaf; they are considered "Class B" travelers (they travel in any area, including in metropolitan areas, but only along routes with which they have been familiarized and trained by an O&M instructor)	Yes, for many years their graduates have independently crossed specifically chosen quiet intersections after first holding up a small stop sign and waiting five seconds to warn drivers. At busier intersections, they get assistance from passersby.
Guide Dog Foundation for the Blind	Accepts students who are hearing impaired, but they must have enough hearing to judge traffic in quiet areas, hear lectures, and have good speech. Has graduated 10 hearing-impaired students during the past five years.	No, if the traveler cannot hear well enough to judge when it is safe to cross, sighted assistance should be obtained, even at quiet, familiar intersections. Traffic training of the dog is geared to elicit an appropriate reaction in an emergency but is not intended to replace the guide dog user's judgment.
Guide Dogs for the Blind	Applicants must have sufficient hearing to judge the flow of traffic and to initiate street crossings independently.	No, the idea that "intelligent disobedience" could be applied to this situation misrepresents the concept. If the dog happens to be facing where it can see an approaching vehicle when the "forward" command is given, it will disobey, but the dog may not be aware of a rapidly approaching car when the command is given.
Guide Dogs of the Desert	Applicants must be able to distinguish vehicular sounds in quiet areas, hear lectures, and receive information from the public. The school has graduated two hearing-impaired students during the past five years.	Although deaf-blind dog guide users have crossed streets independently, the school does not advise students to do it. It would require a dog with special qualities. Possible places where a person with such a dog may be able to cross are quiet, familiar streets, including those with busy parallel streets, but not those with traffic lights. Rural highways with occasional traffic would require a lot of training.

Guiding Eyes for the Blind	The school accepts deaf-blind students, regardless of the amount of remaining hearing or vision they have. An interview in the applicant's home area is required. Although the school is willing to provide room and board for an interpreter if needed, the student must arrange for and pay the interpreter. During the past five years, the school has graduated 66 students who were deaf or hearing impaired.	Yes, certain intersections may be appropriate for independent crossings if they are familiar and if the individual can maintain orientation and direction. For the majority of crossings, soliciting aid is encouraged and practiced.
International Guiding Eyes	If communication can be established, the school will accept deaf-blind students. It graduated three profoundly deaf students when the school had a trainer who could sign.	No, because the person who is deaf-blind would not know when it is safe to give the "forward" command and could be in danger. Before graduating, students who cannot adequately judge traffic conditions must sign a statement that they agree not to cross any street unassisted.
Leader Dogs for the Blind	The school accepts deaf-blind students if their speech is understandable, although it is interested in developing procedures to train students who have no speech. It has graduated five deaf-blind students during the past five years and has two trainers who can sign.	Yes, at quiet streets and at intersections with four-way stop signs. Busy streets or those with a traffic light should not be crossed without assistance.
Pilot Dogs	The school accepts hearing-impaired blind applicants. A home interview determines the applicant's acceptance and dictates the qualities the dog should possess.	The person who is deaf-blind is encouraged to request assistance in crossing streets. Quiet, well-known areas may be negotiated if the user is confident and understands the limits of his or her abilities.
The Seeing Eye	The applicant must be able to judge the flow of traffic. The school routinely accepts hearing-impaired students and graduated one deaf-blind student who was a skilled dog guide user before becoming deaf.	Yes, but street crossings must be done by dog guides with certain characteristics and must be chosen especially for this purpose. Dog guides must not be given this responsibility frequently or they will not be able to handle it.

Southeastern Guide Dogs	Applicants must be able to hear the instructor in a controlled area before training or have a combination of remaining functional hearing and vision. The school prefers that students be able to speak. It has two instructors who can sign. During the past three years, it has graduated 16 deaf or severely hearing impaired blind individuals.	Yes, on special request, dog guides can be trained to cross most streets except rural highways. The school considers rural highways, even those with only occasional traffic, to be the most dangerous areas.

GLOSSARY

Arc of the Cane. The pattern that the cane tip makes as it is moved from left to right. The correct arc for most cane techniques is about an inch wider than the traveler's body.

Assistive Listening Device. A device that enables a person to hear a voice or other sound directly with background noises reduced (see Compton, 1989, in References). Hard-wired and wireless systems are available.

Audible Traffic Signal. A device that is installed at a traffic signal to provide audible output indicating when the signal changes from red to green.

Augmentative Communication Device. A device that produces spoken messages. Messages may be recorded ahead of time and reproduced by pushing a button or may be produced by a speech synthesizer as the words are spelled out on a keyboard.

Communication Book (or Poster). A notebook, paper, poster, or set of cards with symbols of everyday concepts and things (such as a milkshake, toilet, or hairbrush, or happy). Symbols can be visual, tactual, or both. The user points to the symbols to request things, announce information, or express feelings. Often the printed word for each concept appears next to its symbol, so outsiders can understand the meaning of the symbols.

Constant-Contact Cane Technique (sometimes called the slide-slide cane technique). A technique in which the cane is held with the hand centered in front of the body, with the tip sliding along the ground in an arc slightly wider than the person's body. As with the touch technique, the tip is moved in rhythm with the feet; with each step, the tip arrives at the end of the arc that is opposite of the forward foot.

Drop-off. An abrupt drop in the surface of the ground, such as at stairs or curbs.

Drop-off Lesson. A lesson in which the client is intentionally disoriented and must apply orientation techniques to try to determine where he or she is.

Echolocation. The use of reflected sound (including ambient sound) to detect the presence of objects, such as walls, buildings, doors, openings, and people. Proficiency with echolocation can also enable a person to determine the size of a room and whether it is furnished.

Electronic Travel Aid (ETA). Device that detects objects in the environment through the use of reflected sonar, radar, or laser beams. If the device detects an object within its range, it gives off an audible or tactual signal or both. The signals of some ETAs indicate the distance of the object, while others indicate only that there is something within the range of their beam (several ETAs have audible signals that also indicate the surface texture or direction or the object).

Except for the laser cane and the Wheelchair Pathfinder, however, ETAs are not mobility aids. While the person is using the ETA to find objects and openings, he or she also uses a cane or dog for safe travel.

Some ETAs are small and hand held; some are worn over the chest or mounted in glasses; one is encased in a cane; and one is designed to be mounted on wheelchairs, walkers, and scooters. The range in which the ETAs can detect objects varies. Many ETAs have a switch that allows the person to choose either a range of about 12 feet in front of the device or about 4 feet, depending on the situation.

Eccentric Viewing. Looking at something with part of the peripheral vision, rather than the central (that is, looking at something by looking to the side, above, or below the object). It is usually done by people whose central vision is impaired.

Hines Break. A technique that people can use when someone else grabs their arm to guide them. Enables them to disengage their arm smoothly and either take the arm of the guide or withdraw from contact. While pivoting at the waist, the person lets the arm that is being grabbed be pushed forward, then reaches under the arm to hold the top of the other person's wrist and push it forward until the hand lets go of his or her arm.

Kinesthetic Sense. The sensation of bodily position or movement, resulting primarily from the stimulation of sensory nerve endings in muscles, tendons, and joints.

Pager (Vibrating Alerting System). System that alerts people who are deaf or deaf-blind about household or environmental sounds. The user carries or wears a receiver that vibrates when one of the transmitters is activated. Some transmitters are connected directly to telephones, doorbells, smoke alarms, and so forth and others respond to nearby sounds, such as a baby's cry.

Partial Occlusion. The obstruction of part of a person's vision. Placing a tape over the bottom half of clients' eyeglasses allows them to practice using their vision for orientation while noticing information from their canes or other senses.

Relay Service. A service that enables a hearing person who has no TDD and a deaf TDD user to talk to each other over the telephone. It has an operator who has two telephones, one of which is connected to a TDD. Callers give the operator the number of the person with whom they wish to talk. The operator then calls that person and facilitates the communication by reading the message from the TDD user for the hearing person and typing the message from the hearing person into the TDD for the deaf person.

Sighted Guide Technique. A specific technique in which a visually impaired person uses a sighted person as a guide. The visually impaired person holds the arm of the guide just above the elbow, with his or her thumb on the outside, and walks to the side and about a half step behind the guide.

TDD (Telecommunication Device for the Deaf). A device used by deaf people to communicate by telephone. It looks like a small typewriter with a display screen (sometimes also with a paper printout) and has two receptacles in which to place the ends of a telephone receiver. Text that is typed on the keyboard is displayed and converted into a series of beeps and chirps, which can be conveyed through the telephone line and displayed as a message on another TDD.

Square Off. To position one's body in alignment with an object (such as a wall or the edge of a table or carpet) to get a line of direction perpendicular to the object.

Tactile Symbol. A symbol that can be identified by touching it.

Three-Point Touch Technique. A technique that is used to search for a sidewalk or grass on top of the curb while walking along the edge of a street. The person moves the cane in an arc touching first on the side opposite the curb, then touching the edge of the curb, then reaching up over the curb to touch the top. The cane touches the two ends of the arc in rhythm with the feet (the side of the curb is touched while the foot is moving forward).

Touch Cane Technique. A technique in which the cane is held with the hand centered in front of the body and the tip is moved just above the ground in an arc that is slightly wider than the person's body and touches the ground at each end of the arc. The tip touches the ground in rhythm with the feet, being on the side of the arc opposite the forward foot.

Trailing a Wall with the Cane. A technique used to find doors or edges along a wall. While walking near the wall, the person moves the tip of the cane in an arc from left to right, as in the touch cane technique, but when the tip is near the wall, it touches the wall, rather than the ground.

Vibrotactile Device. A small, portable device that transforms sounds into vibrations that can be felt by the person wearing the device (usually on the chest or wrist). Such devices were developed to help deaf people lipread, but they can also enable deaf-blind people to be aware of environmental sounds, such as traffic, dogs' barks, and people's footsteps.

REFERENCES

Baker, C., & Battison, R. (Eds.). (1980). *Sign language and the deaf community*. Silver Spring, MD: National Association of the Deaf.

Barr, M. L. (1974). *The human nervous system* (2nd ed). Hagerstown, MD: Harper & Row.

Battison, R. (1980). Signs have parts: A simple idea. In C. Baker & R. Battison (Eds.), *Sign language and the deaf community* (pp. 35-51). Silver Spring, MD: National Association of the Deaf.

California State Department of Health. (1974). *Leisure time activities for deaf-blind children*. Northridge, CA: Joyce Motion Picture Co.

Canadian National Institute for the Blind (CNIB). (1992). *Functional assessments for work with deaf-blind persons*. Toronto: Author.

Chen, D., & Smith, J. (1992). Developing orientation and mobility skills in students who are multihandicapped and visually impaired. *Re:VIEW, 24*(3), 133-139.

Cokely, D. (1980). Sign language: Teaching, interpreting, and educational policy. In C. Baker & R. Battison (Eds.), *Sign language and the deaf community* (pp. 137-158). Silver Spring, MD: National Association of the Deaf.

Community-based living options for young adults with deaf-blindness. (1987). Sands Point, NY: TAC-Helen Keller National Center.

Compton, Cynthia. (1989). *Assistive listening devices: Doorways to independence*. Washington, DC: Assistive Devices Center, Gallaudet University.

De L'Aune, W. R. (1980). Hearing: Its evolution and ways of compensating for its loss. *Journal of Visual Impairment & Blindness, 74*, 19-23.

DeFiore, E.N., & Silver, R. (1988). A redesigned assistance card for the deaf-blind traveler. *Journal of Visual Impairment & Blindness, 82*, 175–177.

Dinsmore, A. (1959). *Methods of communication with deaf-blind people*. New York: American Foundation for the Blind.

DiPietro, L. (Ed.). (1978). *Guidelines on interpreting for deaf-blind persons*. Washington, DC: Public Service Programs, Gallaudet College.

Duncan, E., Prickett, H., Finkelstein, D., Vernon, M., & Hollingsworth, T. (1988) . *Usher's syndrome: What it is, how to cope, and how to help*. Springfield, IL: Charles C Thomas.

Erting, C. (1980). Sign language and communication between adults and children. In C. Baker & R. Battison (Eds.), *Sign language and the deaf community* (pp. 159-176). Silver Spring, MD: National Association of the Deaf.

Florence, I. J., & LaGrow, S. J. (1989). The use of a recorded message for gaining assistance with street crossings for deaf-blind travelers. *Journal of Visual Impairment & Blindness, 83*, 471–472.

Gee, K., Harrell, R., & Rosenberg, R. (1987). Teaching orientation and mobility skills within and across natural opportunities for travel: A model designed for learners with multiple severe disabilities. In L. Goetz & D. Guess (Eds.), *Innovative program design for individuals with dual sensory impairments* (pp. 127-157). Baltimore, MD: Paul H. Brookes.

Geruschat, D. R. (1980). Orientation and mobility for the low functioning deaf-blind child. *Journal of Visual Impairment & Blindness, 74,* 29-33.

Goetz, L., & Guess, D. (Eds.). (1987). *Innovative program design for individuals with dual sensory impairments.* Baltimore, MD: Paul H. Brookes.

Hoemann, H. W. (1976). *The American Sign Language.* Silver Spring, MD: National Association of the Deaf.

Hultkrantz, A. (1987). *Native religions of North America: The power of visions and fertility.* San Francisco: Harper & Row.

Humphries, T., Padden, C., & O'Rourke, T. J. (1980). *A basic course in American Sign Language.* Silver Spring, MD: T.J. Publishers.

Joffee, Elga. (1991). Orientation and mobility for students with severe visual and multiple impairments: A new perspective. *Journal of Visual Impairment & Blindness, 85,* 211–216.

Johnson, K. (1992, June). *The meaning of community.* Paper presented at the convention of the American Association of the Deaf-Blind, Minneapolis, MN.

Kates, L., & Schein, J. (1980). *A complete guide to communication with deaf-blind persons.* Silver Spring, MD: National Association of the Deaf.

Kinney, R. (1972). *Independent living without sight and hearing.* Winnetka, IL: Hadley School for the Blind.

Kraft, M. E. (1988). Analyzing technological risks in federal regulatory agencies. In M. E. Kraft, & N. J. Vig (Eds.), *Technology and Politics* (pp. 184-207). Durham, NC: Duke University Press.

Lamb, P. (1989). Listen to me—I am human too. *The Deaf-Blind American, 28*(2), 26-27.

Lash, J. P. (1980). *Helen and teacher.* New York: American Foundation for the Blind.

Lawhorn, G. (1991). *On different roads: An autobiography by Geraldine Lawhorn.* New York: Vantage Press.

Lindstrom, J.-I. (1990). Technological solutions for visually impaired people in Sweden. *Journal of Visual Impairment & Blindness, 84,* 513–516.

Lolli, D. A. (1980). Deaf-blind persons. In R. Welsh & B. Blasch, (Eds.), *Foundations of orientation and mobility* (pp. 438-445). New York: American Foundation for the Blind.

Lowrance, W. W. (1976). *Of acceptable risk: Science and the determination of safety.* Los Altos, CA: William Kaufman.

Markowicz, H. (1977). *American Sign Language: Fact and fancy.* Washington, DC: Gallaudet University.

Mendelson, J. H., Kubzansky, P. E., Harrison, R., Siger, L., Leiderman, P. H., Ervin, F. R., Wexler, D., & Solomon, P. (1964). Effects of visual deprivation on imagery experienced by deaf subjects. *Recent Advances in Biological Psychiatry, 6,* chap. 7.

Michaud, M. (1990). Making the difference for deaf-blind travelers in mass transit. In M. Uslan, A. Peck, W. Wiener, & A. Stern (Eds.) *Access to mass transit for blind and visually impaired travelers* (pp. 137-150). New York: American Foundation for the Blind.

Möller, C. (1992, June). *Ears, deafness, and balance.* Paper presented at the convention of the American Association of the Deaf-Blind, Minneapolis, MN.

Murphy, P. (1989, August). *Setting the scene.* Paper presented at the convention of the National Deaf-Blind League, York, England.

Ohlson, S. (1989, August). *Communication with the deaf-blind other than fingerspelling.* Paper presented at the convention of the National Deaf-Blind League, York, England.

Primrose-McGowan, M. (1980, June). *Orientation and mobility training for deaf-blind adults.* Paper presented at Helen Keller Congress, Boston.

Rowland, C., & Stremel-Campbell, K. (1987).Share and share alike: Conventional gestures to emergent language for learners with sensory impairments. In L. Goetz, D. Guess, & K. Stremel-Campbell (Eds.) *Innovative program design for individuals with dual sensory impairments* (pp. 49-75). Baltimore, MD: Paul H. Brookes.

Sauerburger, D. (1987). Using the timing method for limited detection to test the effectiveness of a vibrotactile device for crossing streets by a deaf-blind person. Unpublished manuscript.

Sauerburger, D. (1989). To cross or not to cross: Objective timing methods of assessing street crossings without traffic controls. *RE:view, 21,* 153–161.

Sauerburger, D. (1991, May) Make your own vision impairment simulators. *Newsletter of the DC-Maryland Association for Education and Rehabilitation of the Blind and Visually Impaired,* pp. 5–6.

Sauerburger, D., & Jones, S. (1992). *Corner to corner: Effective ways to solicit aid by deaf-blind people.* Unpublished manuscript.

Signorat, M., & Watson, A. (1981, December). Orientation and mobility training for the multiply handicapped deaf. *Teaching Exceptional Children,* pp. 110–115.

Slade, P. D., & Bentall, R. P. (1988). *Sensory deception: A scientific analysis of hallucination.* Baltimore, MD: Johns Hopkins University Press.

Smithdas, R. J. (1982). *Shared beauty.* New York: Portal Press.

Solomon, P., Kubzansky, P., Leiderman, P. H., Mendelson, J., Trumbull, R., & Wexler, D. (1965). *Sensory deprivation, A symposium held at Harvard Medical School.* Cambridge, MA: Harvard University Press.

Stevens, R. (1980). Education in schools for deaf children. In C. Baker & R. Battison (Eds.), *Sign language and the deaf community* (pp. 177-191). Silver Spring, MD: National Association of the Deaf.

Stiefel, D. H. (1991). *The Madness of Usher's: Coping with vision and hearing loss (Usher's syndrome Type II).* Corpus Christi, TX: The Business of Living Publications.

Strategies for serving deaf-blind clients. (1984). Hot Springs, AR: University of Arkansas.

Suedfeld, P. (1969). Changes in intellectual performance and in susceptibility to influence. In J. Zubek (Ed.), *Sensory deprivation: Fifteen years of research* (pp. 126-166). New York: Meredith Corp.

Trybus, R. (1980). Sign language, power, and mental health. In C. Baker & R. Battison (Eds.), *Sign language and the deaf community.* Silver Spring, MD: National Association of the Deaf.

Vernon, M., & Hicks, W. (1983). A group counseling and educational program for students with Usher's syndrome. *Journal of Visual Impairment & Blindness, 77,* 64–66.

Welsh, R. L. (1980). Psychosocial dimensions. In R. L. Welsh & B. B. Blasch (Eds.), *Foundations of orientation and mobility* (pp. 225-264). New York: American Foundation for the Blind.

Wiener, W. (1980). Audition. In R. L. Welsh & B. B. Blasch (Eds.), *Foundations of orientation and mobility* (pp. 115-185). New York: American Foundation for the Blind.

Woodward, J. (1980). Sociolinguistic research on American Sign Language. In C. Baker & R. Battison (Eds.), *Sign language and the deaf community* (pp. 117-134). Silver Spring, MD: National Association of the Deaf.

Wynne, B. (1987). The deaf-blind population: Etiology and implications for rehabilitation. In *Community-based living options for young adults with deaf-blindness* (pp. 3-23). Sands Point, NY: TAC-Helen Keller National Center.

Yoken, C. (1979). *Living with deaf-blindness*. Washington, DC: National Academy of Gallaudet College.

Zubek, J. P. (Ed.). (1969). *Sensory deprivation: Fifteen years of research*. New York: Meredith Corp.

RESOURCES

A wide variety of organizations disseminate useful information, produce specialized materials, and provide services to benefit persons who are deaf and blind, their families, and the professionals who work with them. This listing contains a representative sampling of the organizations that can offer assistance and information and of the adaptive equipment and other products designed to help people with visual and hearing impairments live independent lives.

SOURCES OF INFORMATION AND SERVICES*

Consumer Organizations

American Association of the Deaf-Blind
814 Thayer Avenue
Silver Spring, MD 20910, USA
(301) 588-6545 (TDD)
Promotes better opportunities and services for deaf-blind people and strives to ensure that a comprehensive, coordinated system of services is accessible to all deaf-blind people, enabling them to achieve their maximum potential through increased independence, productivity, and integration into the community. Publishes *The Deaf-Blind American*.

American Council of the Blind
1155 15th Street, N.W., Suite 720
Washington, DC 20005, USA
(202) 467-5081; (800) 424-8666
Promotes effective participation of blind people in all aspects of society. Provides information and referral, legal assistance, scholarships, advocacy, consultation, and program development assistance. Interest groups include the Deaf-Blind Committee and the Council of Citizens with Low Vision International. Publishes *The Braille Forum*.

Canadian Association of the Deaf
2435 Holly Lane, Suite 205
Ottawa, Ontario K1V 7P2, Canada
(613) 526-4785 (voice/TDD); FAX: (613) 526-4718
Provides deaf persons and representatives of organizations with opportunities to meet. Responsible for educating the government and public on issues concerning deaf persons. Advocates for deaf Canadians. Publishes *Canadian Deaf Advocate* together with the Canadian Cultural Society of the Deaf and the Canadian Deaf Sports Association.

Canadian Council of the Blind
396 Cooper Street, Suite 405
Ottawa, Ontario K2P 2H7, Canada
(613) 567-0311; FAX (613) 567-2728
Provides social, recreation, and blindness prevention programs. Advocates on behalf of blind and visually impaired persons.

*Some materials appearing here and in "Distributors and Manufacturers" were provided by Rustie Rothstein, regional representative, Helen Keller National Center for Deaf-Blind Youths and Adults.

Canadian Cultural Society of the Deaf
House 144
11337 - 61 Avenue
Edmonton, Alberta T6H 1M3, Canada
(403) 436-2599 (TDD); FAX: 403-430-9489
Encourages and facilitates the self-realization of deaf persons to their fullest potential within the general Canadian society; advances the cultural interests of deaf Canadians; encourages research and participation in the arts, humanities, and social sciences; assists in dealing with the differences in sign languages across Canada (Canadian, French, Maritime, and Eskimo); and promotes better understanding between the deaf and hearing communities. Publishes the *Canada Directory of ASL* and *Deaf Heritage in Canada*.

Canadian Deafened Persons Association
c/o CRCHI
310 Elmgrove Avenue
Ottawa, Ontario K1Z 6V1, Canada
(613) 729-6274 (TDD)
Provides a variety of services and programs that include supportive outreach, self-help support groups for late-deafened persons, social activities, and advocacy. Publishes newsletter.

Canadian Hard of Hearing Association
2435 Holly Lane, Suite 205
Ottawa, Ontario K1V 7P2, Canada
(613) 526-1584 (voice); (613) 526-2692 (TDD); FAX: (613) 526-4718
Advocates for hard-of-hearing people in social, educational, and employment environments; lobbies for accessibility. Services also include social activities. Publishes *Listen*.

Canadian National Society of the Deaf-Blind
422 Willowdale Avenue, #405
Toronto, Ontario M2N 5B1, Canada
(416) 480-7417 (voice/TDD)
Promotes the advancement of educational, economic, social, and recreational opportunities for deaf-blind persons; advances public awareness; and advocates for deaf-blind people on the national and provincial government levels so that they may be full participants in Canadian society.

National Association of the Deaf
814 Thayer Avenue
Silver Spring, MD 20910, USA
(301) 587-1788 (voice); (301) 587-1789 (TDD)
Committed to improving the quality of products and services for deaf and hard-of-hearing people. Advocates for legislation for equal access to communication and employment opportunities, has a legal defense fund, public information center, youth programs in professional leadership, and Sign Instructors Guidance Network. Publishes books, pamphlets, videos, *The NAD Broadcaster,* and *The Deaf American*.

National Federation of the Blind
1800 Johnson Street
Baltimore, MD 21230, USA
(410) 659-9314
Strives to improve social and economic conditions of blind persons, evaluates and assists in establishing programs, and provides public education and scholarships. Inter-

est groups include the Committee on the Concerns of the Deaf-Blind. Publishes *The Braille Monitor* and *Future Reflections*.

Self Help for Hard of Hearing People
7800 Wisconsin Avenue
Bethesda, MD 20897, USA
(301) 657-2248 (voice); (301) 657-2249 (TDD)
Promotes awareness of and information about hearing loss, communication, assistive devices, and alternative communication skills through publications, exhibits, and presentations. Publishes *SHHH*.

Resource Agencies

Alexander Graham Bell Association for the Deaf, Inc.
3417 Volta Place, N.W.
Washington, DC 20007, USA
(202) 337-5220 (voice/TDD)
Provides information and public education about hearing loss in children and adults. Publishes *Volta Review*, *Newsounds*, and *Our Kids Magazine*.

American Deafness and Rehabilitation Association
P.O. Box 251554
Little Rock, AR 72225, USA
(501) 663-7074 (voice/TDD)
Promotes and participates in the provision of social and rehabilitation services to deaf people as a partnership with national organizations, local affiliates, professional sections, and individual members. Publishes *Journal of American Deafness and Rehabilitation Association* and *ADARA UPDATE Newsletter*.

American Foundation for the Blind
15 West 16th Street
New York, NY 10011, USA
(212) 620-2000; (800) 232-5463
Provides services to and acts as an information clearinghouse for people who are blind or visually impaired and their families, professionals, organizations, schools, and corporations. Stimulates research to improve services to visually impaired persons; develops and sells adapted products; advocates for services and legislation; maintains the M.C. Migel Memorial Library and the Helen Keller Archives; and publishes books, pamphlets, videos, the *Directory of Services for Blind and Visually Impaired Persons in the United States and Canada*, and the *Journal of Visual Impairment & Blindness*.

American Printing House for the Blind
1839 Frankfort Avenue
Louisville, KY 40206, USA
(502) 895-2405
Produces materials in braille, large print, and on audiocassette; manufactures computer-access equipment, software, and special educational devices for visually impaired persons; maintains an educational research and development program and a reference-catalog service providing information about volunteer-produced textbooks in accessible media.

Arkansas Rehabilitation Research and Training for Persons Who Are Deaf and Hard of Hearing
University of Arkansas
4601 West Markham Street
Little Rock, AR 72205, USA
(501) 686-9691 (voice/TDD)
Focuses on issues affecting the employability of people who are deaf or hard of hearing and provides information about the rehabilitation of those who are served by vocational rehabilitation programs.

Association for Education and Rehabilitation of the Blind and Visually Impaired
206 North Washington Street, Suite 320
Alexandria, VA 22314, USA
(703) 548-1884
Promotes all phases of education and work for blind and visually impaired persons of all ages, strives to expand their opportunities to take a contributory place in society, and disseminates information. Certifies rehabilitation teachers, orientation and mobility specialists, and classroom teachers. Interest groups include the Multihandicapped and Deaf-Blind Division. Publishes *RE:view, AER Report,* and *Job Exchange Monthly.*

Association of Visual Language Interpreters of Canada
11337 61st Avenue
Edmonton, Alberta T6H 1M3, Canada
(403) 430-9442
Advances and promotes high standards for the profession of interpreting. Offers the Canadian Evaluation System, a national certification for ASL/English interpreters. Publishes *AVLIC News.*

The Bicultural Center
5506 Kenilworth Avenue, Suite 100
Riverdale, MD 20737, USA
(301) 699-5226 (voice/TDD)
Disseminates information and promotes public education on interaction of deaf and hearing cultures and fosters acceptance of natural sign languages. Publishes *TBC News.*

Canadian Deaf and Hard of Hearing Forum
2435 Holly Lane, Suite 205
Ottawa, Ontario K1V 7P2, Canada
(613) 526-4867 (voice); (613) 526-2498 (TDD); FAX: (613) 526-4718
Provides a mechanism for information exchange and cooperation among consumers and professionals. Develops structures which allow consumer organizations for deaf and hard-of-hearing persons to participate in discussions of issues to search for solutions.

Canadian Deaf-Blind and Rubella Association
747 Second Avenue East, Suite 4
Owen Sound, Ontario N4K 2G9, Canada
(519) 372-1333 (voice/TDD)
Is committed to ensuring that all deaf-blind persons are provided with optimum services needed to facilitate their integration into Canadian society and economic structures. Promotes the development and implementation of programs such as one-on-one intervention. Publishes *Intervention.*

Canadian Hearing Society
271 Spadina Road
Toronto, Ontario M5R 2V3, Canada
(416) 964-9595 (voice); (416) 964-0023 (TDD); FAX: (416) 964-2066
Provides a wide range of direct services to deaf persons, including audiology, hearing aid programs, assistance with technical devices, employment, vocational rehabilitation, personal counseling, interpreters, sign-language classes, and a program for elderly persons.

Canadian National Institute for the Blind
Deaf-Blind Services
1929 Bayview Avenue
Toronto, Ontario, M4G 3E8, Canada
(416) 480-7417 (voice/TDD)
Provides teaching and facilitation services to enable deaf-blind people to gain and maintain independence and access to information; offers orientation and mobility training, counseling, rehabilitation teaching, and English literacy services to deaf-blind people.

Convention of American Instructors of the Deaf
National Technical Institute for the Deaf
c/o Rochester Institute of Technology
JBJ-2264
P.O. Box 9887
Rochester, NY 14623-0887, USA
(716) 475-6201 (voice/TDD)
Promotes professional development, communication, and information among educators of deaf individuals and other interested people. Publishes *American Annals of the Deaf* and *News 'n Notes*.

Deaf-Blind Program
Perkins School for the Blind
175 North Beacon Street
Watertown, MA 02172, USA
(617) 924-3434
Provides direct support services to deaf-blind children, their families, and the professionals who work with them. Provides leadership and advocacy programs for deaf-blind people and collaborates with other organizations to improve their quality of life.

Gallaudet University
800 Florida Avenue, N.E.
Washington, DC 20002-3695, USA
(202) 651-5000 (voice/TDD)
Serves deaf and hard-of-hearing individuals through education, research, and public service and disseminates information. Operates the Hearing-Vision Impaired Program, National Information Center on Deafness, National Center for Law and Deafness, Research Institute, and Media Distribution Center. Its university press publishes books, pamphlets, and videos.

Hadley School for the Blind
700 Elm Street
Winnetka, IL 60093-0299, USA
(708) 446-8111
Provides tuition-free home studies in academic subjects as well as vocational and technical areas, personal enrichment, parent/child issues, compensatory rehabili-

tation education, and bible study. Rehabilitation courses include topics such as braille, abacus and, for deaf-blind adults, independent living without sight and hearing.

Helen Keller National Center for Deaf-Blind Youths and Adults
111 Middle Neck Road
Sands Point, NY 11050-1299, USA
(516) 944-8900 (voice/TDD)
The national center and its 10 regional offices provide diagnostic evaluations, comprehensive vocational and personal adjustment training, and job preparation and placement for people who are deaf-blind from every state and territory. Provides technical assistance and training to those who work with deaf-blind people. Publishes *The Nat-Cent News*, *National Parent Newsletter*, and *TAC Newsletter*.

Hilton-Perkins National Program
Perkins School for the Blind
175 North Beacon Street
Watertown, MA 02172, USA
(617) 924-3434
Improves the quality of life for underserved, multiply disabled blind and deaf-blind children and their families. Determines program needs and provides direct and support services to children, their families, and professionals in the United States and developing countries around the world. Provides leadership and advocacy for programs for multiply disabled blind and deaf-blind children.

Mississippi State University Rehabilitation Research and Training Center on Blindness and Low Vision
P.O. Drawer 6189
Mississippi State, MS 39762, USA
(601) 625-2001
Conducts a variety of applied research projects concerning blindness, visual impairment, and deaf-blindness. Conducts in-service training programs for state agencies, national training conferences, and research forums. Publishes monographs on related subjects and a newsletter, *Worksight*.

National Coalition on Deaf-Blindness
175 North Beacon Street
Watertown, MA 02172, USA
(617) 972-7347; FAX: (617) 923-8076
Advocates on behalf of the interests of deaf-blind children and adults via maintaining contact with legislators and policy-making agencies. Comprised of national organizations that have an interest in services to deaf-blind people and individual members, including professionals, parents, and consumers interested in influencing such services.

National Technical Institute for the Deaf
Rochester Institute of Technology, Public Information Office
One Lomb Memorial Drive
P.O. Box 9887
Rochester, NY 14623, USA
(716) 475-6400 (voice); (716) 475-2181 (TDD)
Provides technological postsecondary education to deaf and hard-of-hearing students. Disseminates informational materials and instructional videotapes on deafness and related areas. Publishes *NTID Focus*.

Registry of Interpreters for the Deaf
8719 Colesville Road, Suite 310
Silver Spring, MD 20910-3919, USA
(301) 608-0050 (voice/TDD)
Certifies interpreters and provides information on interpreting to the general public. Interest groups include the Special Interest Group Focusing on Deaf-Blind Issues. Publishes *Views.*

RP Foundation Fighting Blindness
1401 Mt. Royal Avenue
Baltimore, MD 21217-4245, USA
(800) 683-5555; (410) 225-9409 (voice); (410) 225-9400 (TDD)
Strives to discover the cause, prevention, and treatment of retinitis pigmentosa. Main office and 60 affiliates in the United States are involved in public education, information and referral, workshops, research, national registry of patients, and fundraising. Publishes *Fighting Blindness News.*

TASH (The Association for Persons with Severe Handicaps)
11201 Greenwood Avenue North
Seattle, WA 98133, USA
(206) 361-8870; (206) 316-0113 (TDD); FAX: (206) 361-9208
Advocates for quality education for persons with disabilities; advocates for the rights of persons with disabilities in legal proceedings; disseminates information; maintains library; bestows awards.

TRACES (Teaching Research Assistance to Children Experiencing Sensory Impairments)
Northwestern Oregon State College
345 North Monmouth Avenue
Monmouth, OR 97361, USA
(503) 838-8391; (503) 838-2256 (TDD); FAX: (503) 838-8150
Provides technical assistance to all state and multistate deaf-blind projects serving children who are deaf-blind. Conducts needs assessments and delivers assistance in a variety of forms with a focus on improving the quality of placements and services for deaf-blind children.

Vestibular Disorders Association
P.O. Box 4467
Portland, OR 97208-4467, USA
(503) 229-7705; FAX: (503) 229-8064
Enhances a support network for people with dizziness and balance disorders; provides information, educates the public, and supports research and clinical activities on vestibular disorders and related topics. Publishes *On the Level.*

Dog Guide Schools

Canadian Guide Dogs for the Blind
4120 Rideau Valley Drive North
Manotick, ON KOA 2N0, Canada
(613) 692-7777

Canine Vision Canada
c/o Lions Foundation of Canada
P.O. Box 907
Oakville, ON L6J 5E8, Canada
(416) 842-2891

Eye Dog Foundation for the Blind, Inc.
512 North Larchmont Boulevard
Los Angeles, CA 90004, USA
(213) 626-3370 or (213) 468-8856

Eye of the Pacific Guide Dogs and Mobility Services, Inc.
747 Amana Street, #407
Honolulu, HI 96814, USA
(808) 941-1088

Fidelco Guide Dog Foundation, Inc.
P.O. Box 142
Bloomfield, CN 06002, USA
(203) 243-5200

Foundation Mira
1820 Rang Nord Oest
Sainte-Madeleine, Quebec PQ JOH 1SO, Canada
(514) 795-3725

Guide Dog Foundation for the Blind, Inc.
371 East Jericho Turnpike
Smithtown, NY 11787-2976, USA
(516) 265-2121; (800) 548-4337

Guide Dogs for the Blind, Inc.
P.O. Box 151200
San Rafael, CA 94915-1200, USA
(415) 499-4000

Guide Dogs of the Desert, Inc.
P.O. Box 1692
Palm Springs, CA 92263, USA
(619) 329-6257

Guiding Eyes for the Blind, Inc.
611 Granite Springs Road
Yorktown Heights, NY 10598, USA
(914) 245-4024

International Guiding Eyes, Inc.
13445 Glenoaks Boulevard
Sylmar, CA 91342, USA
(213) 362-5834

Leader Dogs for the Blind
P.O. Box 5000
Rochester MI 48307, USA
(313) 651-9011

Pilot Dogs, Inc.
625 West Town Street
Columbus, OH 43215, USA
(614) 221-6367

The Seeing Eye, Inc.
P.O. Box 375
Morristown, NJ 07960, USA
(201) 539-4425

Southeastern Guide Dogs, Inc.
4210 77th Street East
Palmetto, FL 34221, USA
(813) 729-5665

EQUIPMENT AND MATERIALS

The addresses and telephone numbers of manufacturers and distributors of the products described in this section are listed under "Distributors and Manufacturers."

Buttons for Identification

Buttons to be worn on clothing to identify the wearer's visual and hearing impairments can be custom-ordered from any button-manufacturing company; a limited supply is available from the *Helen Keller National Center for Deaf-Blind Youths and Adults*.

Communication Devices

Assistive Listening Devices

Audex Home TV Listening Systems and Wide-Area Systems: Wireless infrared systems, which transmit sounds to the listener's receiver via infrared signals that are contained within the walls of a room. The transmitter can be connected to a television, can use a microphone, or can be installed in a public-address system.
Manufacturer: *Audex*.

Audex SounDirector: Hard-wired system that connects amplified sounds directly to the listener's receiver with a transmitter that uses a microphone.
Manufacturer: *Audex*.

Companion: Wireless FM system, which transmits sounds to the listener's receiver via FM signals that can pass through walls. The transmitter uses a microphone worn by the speaker.
Manufacturer: *Audio Enhancement*.

Easy Listener FM System: Wireless FM system, which transmits sounds to the listener's receiver via FM signals that can pass through walls. The transmitter can be installed in a public-address system or attached to a microphone.
Manufacturer: *Phonic Ear*.

Pocket Talker: Hard-wired system that connects amplified sounds directly to the listener's receiver with a transmitter that can use a microphone or be connected to a television.
Manufacture: *Williams Sound.*

Wireless Sound Enhancement System: Wireless FM system, which transmits sounds to the listener's receiver via FM signals that can pass through walls. The transmitter uses a microphone.
Manufacturer: *Telex.*

Face-to-Face

Alphabet Plate: Plastic board 4 inches by 6.5 inches with raised-line print letters and numerals. No longer manufactured, but still in limited supply.
Distributor: *Helen Keller National Center for Deaf-Blind Youths and Adults.*

Alva Braille Carrier: A portable, electronic communication device. One person types on a braille keyboard that transfers to a print display on the opposite side; another person types on a QWERTY (i.e., typewriter-like) keyboard, and the message comes out on a 40-cell braille display on the other side. The device can also function as a notetaker or as a terminal for a computer.
Manufacturer: *HumanWare, Inc.*

Braille Alphabet Card: Cards with braille letters indicated for each printed letter of the alphabet. Laminated cards can be made by brailling the alphabet onto a see-through Braillabel sheet and adhering the sheet to a card on which the print letters appear above each corresponding braille letter. Braille alphabet cards are available from the *American Foundation for the Blind*, the *American Printing House for the Blind*, and *Howe Press*. Braillabels are available from the *American Thermoform Corporation.*

Brailtalk: A small plastic board that folds in half and that has raised-line print letters and numerals with braille beneath them.
Distributor: *American Foundation for the Blind*

Mountbatten Brailler: An electronic braille-writing device which can be connected to a printer and a computer keyboard. When a person types on the computer keyboard or the Mountbatten Brailler keyboard, the message is printed on paper in inkprint, in Grade II braille, or both. The device can also be used as a notetaker or computer terminal.
Manufacturer: *HumanWare, Inc.*

TeleBraille II: See "Telephone."

Teletouch: A portable mechanical device on which one person types on a keyboard while the other person feels the letters using a single braille cell output.
Distributor: *American Foundation for the Blind.*

Telephone

Amplifier handsets and snap-on amplifiers are available for telephones from *HARC Mercantile, Nationwide Flashing Signal Systems*, and *AT&T Phone Stores* (distributors are located throughout the United States).

AT&T 2830 Printing TDD: Print-out for TDD can be 24, 20, or 12 characters per line.
Distributors: *HARC Mercantile, Nationwide Flashing Signal Systems, AT&T Phone Stores* (distributors are located throughout the United States).

Krown TDD Memory Printer: Print-out for TDD can be 24, 20, or 12 characters per line.
Manufacturer and distributor: *KRI Communication/Krown Research.*
Distributor: *HARC Mercantile.*

Large Visual Display: Device that makes characters ten times as large as those on a standard TDD display, with a variety of available lens colors.
Manufacturer and distributor: *Ultratec.*
Distributors: *HARC Mercantile, Maxi-Aids.*

Infotouch: Device consisting of a braille printer, TDD modem, data detector, and special connector (with an answering machine). TDD signals coming over the telephone are printed in braille on paper, and the user types the response on the TDD keyboard.
Manufacturer: *Enabling Technologies Company.*

TeleBraille II: Device that is connected to a special TDD to provide a row of refreshable braille cells. Messages are typed on the TDD keyboard or are received over the telephone from another TDD and are converted into braille and appear in print on the TDD screen. Can be used for telephone and face-to-face communication to spell out braille and print messages.
Manufacturer: *TeleSensory Systems.*

Voice-prepared Messages

Attention-Getter: Device that produces from one to 12 programmable prepared voice messages for communicating with the public, either personally or over the phone.
Manufacturer: *Companion Products International.*

Mini Talking Card Reader: Device that has the same features as Voxcom (see *Voxcom*).
Distributor: *Crestwood Company.*

Speaking Dynamically: Software for the Macintosh PowerBook laptop computer that provides pictures and symbols with speech output. To activate the individually prepared message, the person can use the keyboard, the cursor, or a switch.
Developer: *Mayer-Johnson Company.*

Tape-A-Message Mike: Tape recorder shaped like a microphone that can record and play back one 15-second continuous loop-taped message.
Distributor: *Crestwood Company.*

VOIS: Portable instrument the size of a computer keyboard that provides speech output for messages typed into the keyboard.
Manufacturer: *Phonic Ear.*

Voxcom: Device for producing voice-prepared messages, which includes reusable magnetic recording tapes and a special cassette recorder that can record or play back the messages on the tapes. The tapes are pressure sensitive and are traditionally used by hearing people to label items such as clothes and records. They can also be fastened to cards to store prerecorded messages to communicate with the public.
Distributors: *American Foundation for the Blind, LS&S Group, Maxi-Aids.*

Communication Books and Cards

Cards: Pocket-sized cards printed on both sides with messages designed for deaf-blind people to solicit aid or communicate with the public.
Developers: *Helen Keller National Center for Deaf-Blind Youths and Adults* and *Volunteers for the Visually Handicapped.*

Object-Picture Talk Board: Three-dimensional replicas of common items that have accompanying pictures and are mounted on a board.
Developer: *Crestwood Company.*

Picture Communication Symbols: Pictures made with easy-to-see line drawings on cards, stickers, or books; sheet protectors and books of various sizes hold and display individually selected drawings.
Developer: *Mayer-Johnson Company.*

Picture Prompt System: Laminated cards with pictures of common items and activities, including cards for deaf-blind persons to use as shopping lists or for recipes.
Developer: *Attainment Company.*

Talking Pictures Kit and Passport System: Cards that illustrate items and activities and are used by deaf-blind persons to interact in the community or to communicate daily needs. Pictures can be stored and displayed in vinyl envelopes on rings, in books, or on boards.
Developer: *Crestwood Company.*

Raised-line Drawing Materials

Hi Marks: Fluorescent orange paste applied with a tube to create raised lines, used for labeling and making objects.
Distributors: *American Foundation for the Blind, Maxi-Aids, LS&S Group.*

Raised-Line Drawing Kit: Kit with plastic sheets, a soft pad on which to place the sheet while drawing, and a stylus for making lines that are embossed as they are drawn.
Distributors: *American Foundation for the Blind, Howe Press, Maxi-Aids.*

Raised Writing Ink: Fast-drying material used to draw raised lines and letters.
Distributor: *SENSE-SATIONS.*

Stereocopier: Machine using special paper to make copies of print letters or drawings into raised-line letters or drawings.
Manufacturer: *SIH Laromedel I Solna.*

Systems for Reading Printed Material

Closed-Circuit Television (CCTV): Video magnification system to enlarge print. Most models have a monitor and small camera suspended above a platform on which the user places the book, newspaper, or other material that he or she wishes to see enlarged. Most can switch the display from dark letters on a white background to white letters on a dark background.
Manufacturers and distributors: *HumanWare, LS&S Group, Optelec, TeleSensory Systems.*

Optacon: A portable reading system that converts the image of a print letter or symbol into an enlarged vibrating tactile form that can be felt with one's finger.
Manufacturer: *TeleSensory Systems.*

Electronic Travel Aids with Tactile Output

Laser Cane: Cane that uses two lasers; one detects objects that are straight ahead and the other detects objects that are above the cane (in front of the face). Two tactile stimulators under the finger vibrate when an object is within the range of the lasers.
Manufacturer: *Nurion Industries.*

Mowat Sensor: Small, hand-held device vibrates when an object is in its beam. Vibrations are faster when closer objects are detected; a switch can limit its range to 4 feet or extend it to 12 feet.
Manufacturer: *HumanWare.*

Pathsounder: Electronic travel aid that is mounted on the chest with a neck strap. The range is usually set so that if an object is detected within 6 feet, the entire device vibrates and gives an audible signal; if the object is within 2.5 feet, the neck strap also vibrates.
Manufacturer: *Lindsay Russell.*

Polaron: Small device that can be hand held or mounted around the neck. It will either vibrate or give an audible signal when an object is in its path. It vibrates faster when an object is closer but gives a strong vibration when it first encounters an object. A switch enables the user to choose a range of detection of 4, 12, or 16 feet.
Manufacturer: *Nurion Industries.*

Wheelchair Pathfinder: Electronic travel aid consisting of two devices that are attached to a wheelchair, walker, or scooter. They alert the user to the presence of objects that are within either 4 or 8 feet in front and 1 foot to the side, and to the presence of drop-offs within 4 feet ahead. The drop-off must be 3 inches or higher to be detected. Either auditory or vibrating signals are provided.
Manufacturer: *Nurion Industries.*

Pagers (Vibrating Alerting Systems)

Knock Sensor: Portable transmitter that can be attached to the inside of any door and activates the receiver or a flashing light when someone knocks.
Manufacturer: *Silent Call Corporation.*

Omni Page Receiver: Receiver that can be coupled with a single transmitter and vibrates when the transmitter is activated within a range of 400 feet of the receiver.
Manufacturer: *Silent Call Corporation.*

Personal Alert System: Vibrating alerting system in which the receiver is clipped to the persons's clothing or is carried. Transmitters include a portable smoke detector, a transmitter for the telephone, a portable sound monitor, a pager, and a doorbell

transmitter. When the receiver vibrates, the person can look at a row of lights on the receiver to know which transmitter is activated.
Manufacturer: *Silent Call Corporation.*

Shake-Up: A portable smoke detector that transmits to a receiver that in turn activates a bed vibrator or strobe light.
Manufacturer: *Sonic Alert.*

Tactile Communicator: Alerting system with a transmitter that can connect with as many as five household devices or sound sources. On the receiver, different vibratory signals indicate which device is activated; a smoke alarm overrides the other signals. The transmitter also has a call button that can be used to tap out coded messages to the user.
Manufacturer: *Silent Call Corporation*

Vibra-Call: An adaptation of the *Personal Alert System* for deaf-blind people. It has a row of four buttons labeled in braille, each of which is associated with a different transmitter (doorbell, telephone, and so on). When the receiver vibrates, the person can push each button until it vibrates again, indicating which transmitter was activated.
Manufacturer: *Silent Call Corporation.*

Sun and Glare Shields

Corning Glare-Control Lenses: Prescribed eyeglasses for people with light sensitivity. Five filter levels available.
Manufacturer: *Corning Medical Optics.*

NoIR and UVShields: Sunglasses with chemical absorbers to regulate the amount of light transmitted. Some have side and top shields.
Manufacturer: *NoIR Medical Technologies.*

Telecaptions with Braille Output

Braille Telecaptioning System: A device that transforms telecaptions, or television subtitles for deaf viewers, into braille.
Distributor: *Dewtronics.*

Traffic Signals with Tactile and Auditory Output

Audio Tactile Pedestrian Detector: Pedestrian push-button walk signal designed for people who are visually impaired. The user pushes the button, which provides tactile as well as auditory output during the signal to walk.
Manufacturer: *AWA Traffic and Information Systems.*

Vibrotactile Devices

TACTAID II+ and TACTAID 7: Devices that vibrate when they detect sounds of 200 to 7,000 Hz. They can be strapped to the wrist or chest. The TACTAID 7 has seven channels and the TACTAID II+ has two channels, each of which respond to a different frequency range.
Manufacturer: *Audiological Engineering Corporation.*

DISTRIBUTORS AND MANUFACTURERS

American Foundation for the Blind
Product Center
100 Enterprise Place
P.O. Box 7044
Dover, DE 19903-7044, USA
(800) 829-0500; (302) 677-0200; FAX: (800) 676-3299

American Printing House for the Blind
P.O. Box 6085
1839 Frankfort Avenue
Louisville, KY 40206, USA
(502) 895-2405; FAX: (502) 895-1509

American Thermoform Corporation
2311 Travers Avenue
City of Commerce, CA 90040, USA
(213) 723-9021; FAX: (213) 728-8877

Attainment Company, Inc.
P.O. Box 930160
504 Commerce Parkway
Verona, WI 53593-0160, USA
(800) 327-4269; FAX: (608) 845-8040

Audex
713 North 4th Street
Longview, TX 75601, USA
(800) 237-0716 (voice/TDD); FAX: (903) 753-9546

Audio Enhancement
1748 West 12600 South
Riverton, UT 84065, USA
(800) 383-9362 (voice/TDD); (801) 254-9263 (voice/TDD); FAX: (801) 254-3802

Audiological Engineering Corporation
35 Medford Street
Somerville, MA 02143, USA
(800) 283-4601 (voice); (800) 955-7204 (TDD); FAX: (617) 666-5228

AWA Traffic and Information Systems
P.O. Box 174, Mitcham VIC 3132
Unit 5, 27 Thornton Crescent, Mitcham
Victoria 3132, Australia
61-3-873-4488; FAX: 02-870-4020

Companion Products International
P.O. Box G
Milford, PA 18337-0208, USA
(800) 258-6423 (voice/TDD); (717) 686-4713 (voice/TDD); FAX: (717) 686-4718

Corning Medical Optics, MP 21-2
North American Optical

Corning, Inc.
Corning, NY 14831, USA
(607) 974-7417; FAX: (607) 974-7088

Crestwood Company
6625 North Sidney Place
Milwaukee, WI 53209, USA
(414) 352-5678; FAX: (414) 352-5679

Dewtronics
987 Via Amorosa
Arnold, MD 21012, USA
(410) 647-0769

Enabling Technologies Company
3102 S.E. Jay Street
Stuart, FL 34997, USA
(407) 283-4817; FAX: (407) 220-2920

HARC Mercantile, Ltd.
Box 3055
Kalamazoo, MI 49003-3055, USA
(800) 445-9968 (voice/TDD); (616) 381-2219 (TDD); (616) 381-0177 (voice); FAX: (616) 381-3614

Helen Keller National Center for Deaf-Blind Youths and Adults
111 Middle Neck Road
Sands Point, NY 11050, USA
(516) 944-8900 (voice/TDD); FAX: (516) 944-7302

Howe Press
Perkins School for the Blind
175 North Beacon Street
Watertown, MA 02172-2790, USA
(617) 924-3490; FAX: (617) 926-2027

HumanWare, Inc.
6245 King Road
Loomis, CA 95650, USA
(916) 652-7253; FAX: (916) 652-7296

KRI Communication, Inc./Krown Research
129 Sheldon Street
El Segundo, CA 90245, USA
Outside California: (800) 833-4968 (voice/TDD); (310) 322-3202 (voice/TDD); FAX: (310) 322-4985

Lindsay Russell
100 Memorial Drive, #11-22B
Cambridge, MA 02142, USA
(617) 547-0819

LS&S Group
P.O. Box 673

Northbrook, IL 60065, USA
(800) 468-4789; FAX: (708) 498-1482

Maxi-Aids
P.O. Box 3209
Farmingdale, NY 11735, USA
(800) 522-6294; FAX: (516) 752-0689

Mayer-Johnson Company
P.O. Box 1579
Solana Beach, CA 92075-1579, USA
(619) 481-2489; FAX: (619) 259-5726

Nationwide Flashing Signal Systems
8120 Fenton Street
Silver Spring, MD 20910, USA
(301) 589-6671 (voice); (301) 589-6670 (TDD); FAX: (301) 589-5153

NoIR Medical Technologies
P.O. Box 159
South Lyon, MI 48178, USA
(800) 521-9746

Nurion Industries
Three Station Square
Paoli, PA 19301, USA
(215) 640-2345; FAX: (215) 647-2216

Optelec, Inc.
6 Lyberty Way
P.O. Box 729
Westford, MA 01886, USA
(800) 828-1056; (508) 392-0707; FAX: (508) 692-6073

Phonic Ear
3880 Cypress Drive
Petaluma, CA 94954-7600, USA
(800) 227-0735 (voice/TDD); (707) 769-1110 (voice/TDD), FAX: (707) 769-9624

SENSE-SATIONS
Associated Services for the Blind
921 Walnut Street
Philadelphia, PA 19107, USA
(215) 627-3304

SIH Laromedel I Solna
Tomtebodavagen 11
S-171 64 Solna, Sweden
08-736-0140

Silent Call Corporation
P.O. Box 868
Clarkston, MI 48347-0868, USA
(800) 572-5227 (voice/TDD); (313) 673-0221 (voice/TDD); FAX: (313) 673-5442

Sonic Alert
1750 West Hamlin Road
Rochester Hills, MI 48309, USA
(313) 656-3110 (voice/TDD); FAX: (313) 656-8347

TeleSensory Systems, Inc.
455 North Bernardo Avenue
P.O. Box 7455
Mountain View, CA 94039, USA
(800) 227-8418; (415) 960-0920; FAX: (415) 969-9064

Telex
9600 Aldrich Avenue South
Minneapolis, MN 55420, USA
(800) 328-3120; (612) 884-4051; FAX: (800) 323-0498

Ultratec
450 Science Drive
Madison, WI 53711-1056, USA
(608) 238-5400 (voice/TDD); FAX: (608) 238-3008

Volunteers for the Visually Handicapped
8720 Georgia Avenue
Silver Spring, MD 20910, USA
(301) 589-0894 (voice/TDD)

Williams Sound
10399 West 70th Street
Eden Prairie, MN 55344, USA
(612) 943-2252 (voice/TDD); FAX: (612) 943-2174

INDEX

ABOUT THE AUTHOR

Dona Sauerburger has been an orientation and mobility instructor at state rehabilitation agencies, private agencies, and schools for the last 20 years, including three years as orientation and mobility specialist for Family Service Foundation's Institute on Deaf-Blindness in Lanham, Maryland. In addition, she has given numerous presentations throughout the United States on issues related to working with people who are deaf-blind.

The mission of the American Foundation for the Blind (AFB) is to enable persons who are blind or visually impaired to achieve equality of access and opportunity that will ensure freedom of choice in their lives. AFB accomplishes this mission by taking a national leadership role in the development and implementation of public policy and legislation, informational and educational programs, diversified products, and quality services. Among the services it delivers, AFB maintains a national hotline to provide information and assistance to callers. The hotline number is 1-800-232-5463; it is in operation Mondays through Fridays, 8:30 a.m. to 4:30 p.m. EST or EDT.

∞

It is the policy of the American Foundation for the Blind to use in the first printing of its books acid-free paper that meets the ANSI Z39.48 Standard. The infinity symbol that appears above indicates that the paper in this printing meets that standard.